WHO Health Evidence Network synthesis report 65

What is the evidence on the methods, frameworks and indicators used to evaluate health literacy policies, programmes and interventions at the regional, national and organizational levels?

Gillian Rowlands | Anita Trezona | Siân Russell | Maria Lopatina | Jürgen Pelikan | Michael Paasche-Orlow | Oxana Drapkina | Anna Kontsevaya | Kristine Sørensen

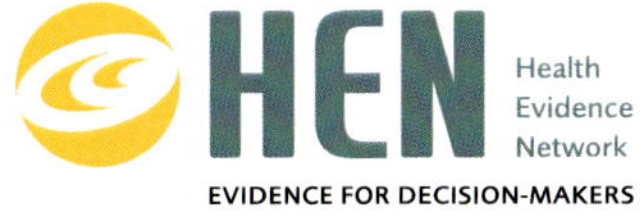

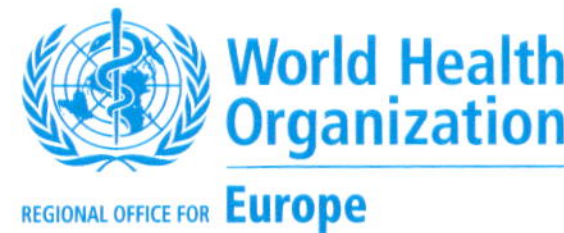

Abstract

Although health literacy has long been a focus of attention in the WHO European Region, survey evidence in 2011 of eight Member States indicated that more than 47% of the adult population had suboptimal personal health literacy. Initiatives to prioritize health literacy in public policies include the WHO Shanghai Declaration, Health 2020, the European policy framework that supports action across government and society for health and well-being and the Health Evidence Network report on health literacy policies in the WHO European Region. This review identifies evidence on the methods, frameworks, measurement instruments, domains and indicators used to evaluate health literacy policies, programmes and interventions at all levels. Limited evidence was found on evaluation of national policies and programmes, but local programmes and interventions have been measured using quantitative, qualitative and mixed-methods approaches. Policy considerations include the development of frameworks and indicators covering a range of domains to enable consistent and comparable population monitoring and evaluations to determine the impact and effectiveness of national policies and programmes.

Keywords

HEALTH LITERACY, HEALTH LITERACY RESPONSIVENESS, HEALTH EDUCATION, HEALTH PROMOTION, HEALTH COMMUNICATION, PROGRAMME EVALUATION

Address requests about publications of the WHO Regional Office for Europe to:

Publications
WHO Regional Office for Europe
UN City, Marmorvej 51
DK-2100 Copenhagen Ø, Denmark

Alternatively, complete an online request form for documentation, health information, or for permission to quote or translate, on the Regional Office website (http://www.euro.who.int/pubrequest).

ISSN 2227-4316
ISBN 978 92 890 5432 4

Suggested citation. WHO Health Evidence Network synthesis report 65. What is the evidence on the methods, frameworks and indicators used to evaluate health literacy policies, programmes and interventions at the regional, national and organizational levels? Copenhagen: WHO Regional Office for Europe; 2019. Licence: CC BY-NC-SA 3.0 IGO.

Cataloguing-in-Publication (CIP) data. CIP data are available at http://apps.who.int/iris.

Printed in Luxembourg

CONTENTS

- Abbreviations iv
- Contributors v
- Summary viii
- 1. Introduction 1
  - 1.1 Background 1
  - 1.2 Methodology 6
- 2. Results 7
  - 2.1 General features of the studies 7
  - 2.2 Evaluation frameworks and logic models 9
  - 2.3 Methods 11
  - 2.4 Measurement domains and indicators 20
  - 2.5 Partnerships and coordination for health literacy measurement 24
  - 2.6 Facilitators and barriers to health literacy measurement 26
  - 2.7 Resources and scalability 29
  - 2.8 Evaluation of health literacy in the WHO European Region 29
- 3. Discussion 31
  - 3.1 Strengths and limitations of this review 31
  - 3.2 Methodological challenges for health literacy measurement 31
  - 3.3 National and regional evaluation and monitoring 33
  - 3.4 Measurement of organizational health literacy responsiveness 34
  - 3.5 Policy considerations 35
- 4. Conclusions 36
- References 37
- Annex 1. Search strategy 52
- Annex 2. Relevant health literacy concepts 61
- Annex 3. Characteristics of health literacy instruments 65

ABBREVIATIONS

AAHLS	All Aspects of Health Literacy Scale
e-HEALS	e-Health Literacy Scale
HeLLO Tas!	self-assessment checklist for an organization's health literacy
HEN	Health Evidence Network
HLQ	Health Literacy Questionnaire
HLS-EU	European Health Literacy Survey
MiMi	With Migrants for Migrants – Intercultural Health in Germany (programme)
M-POHL Network	WHO Action Network on Population and Organizational Health Literacy
ÖPGK	Austrian Platform for Health Literacy
SILS	Single Item Literacy Screener
STOFHLA	Short Test of Functional Health Literacy in Adults

CONTRIBUTORS

This report has been produced with the financial assistance of the Federal Ministry of Health, Germany. The views expressed herein can in no way be taken to reflect the official opinion of the Federal Ministry of Health, Germany.

Authors

Gillian Rowlands
Professor of General Practice, Newcastle University, Newcastle, United Kingdom

Anita Trezona
Managing Director, Trezona Consulting Group, Melbourne, Australia

Siân Russell
Postdoctoral Research Associate, Institute of Health and Society, Newcastle University, Newcastle, United Kingdom

Maria Lopatina
Researcher, National Medical Research Centre for Preventive Medicine under the Ministry of Health of the Russian Federation, Moscow, Russia Federation

Jürgen Pelikan
Professor Emeritus, University of Vienna and Head of the WHO Collaborating Centre on Health Promotion in Hospitals and Health Care at the Austrian Public Health Institute, Vienna, Austria

Michael Paasche-Orlow
Professor of Medicine, Boston University School of Medicine, Boston Medical Centre, Boston, United States of America

Oxana Drapkina
Director, National Medical Research Centre for Preventive Medicine under the Ministry of Health of the Russian Federation, Moscow, Russia Federation

Anna Kontsevaya
Deputy Director of Science and Analytics, National Medical Research Centre for Preventive Medicine under the Ministry of Health of the Russian Federation, Moscow, Russia Federation

Kristine Sørensen
Director, Global Health Literacy Academy, Risskov, Denmark

Peer reviewers

Sabrina Kurtz-Rossi
Assistant Professor, Tufts University School of Medicine; Principal, Kurtz-Rossi & Associates; Director, Health Literacy Leadership Institute; and Secretary General, International Health Literacy Association, Boston, United States of America

Kirsten McCaffery
Professor, School of Public Health, University of Sydney, Sydney, Australia

Danielle M. Muscat
Postdoctoral Research Fellow, Sydney Health Literacy Laboratory, School of Public Health, University of Sydney, Sydney, Australia

Acknowledgements

The authors wish to acknowledge the following people for sharing their knowledge and expertise as part of the expert enquiry: Wagida A. Anwar, Palle Bager, Anne Leonora Blaakilde, Shyam Sundar Budhathoki, Valeria Caponnetto, Claudia Cianfrocca, Xavier Debussche, Bodil Helbech Hansen, Sarah Hosking, Qaiser Iqbal, Hirono Ishikawa, Aulia Iskandarsyah, Zdeněk Kučera, Angela Y. M. Leung, Diane Levin-Zamir, Miroslava Líšková, Julien Mancini, Maria Mares, Katarinne Lima Moraes, Alicia O'Cathain, Orkan Okan, Pinar Okyay, Richard Osborne, Leena Paakkari, Adèle Perrin, Jany Rademakers, Alexandra Rouquette, Lidia Segura Garcia, Sandra Staffieri, Lærke Steenberg Olesen, Eric Van Ganse, Josefin Wångdahl, Anne Wingstrand and Ling Zhang.

Editorial team, WHO Regional Office for Europe

Division of Noncommunicable Diseases and Promoting Health through the Life-course

Bente Mikkelsen, Director
Anastasia Koylyu, Technical Officer

Health Evidence Network (HEN) editorial team

Kristina Mauer-Stender, Acting Director
Tanja Kuchenmüller, Editor in Chief
Ryoko Takahashi, Series Editor
Tyrone Reden Sy, Technical Officer
Krista Kruja, Consultant
Jane Ward, Technical Editor

The HEN Secretariat is part of the Division of Information, Evidence, Research and Innovation at the WHO Regional Office for Europe. HEN synthesis reports are commissioned works that are subjected to international peer review, and the contents are the responsibility of the authors. They do not necessarily reflect the official policies of the Regional Office.

SUMMARY

The issue

Health literacy can be defined as the capacity of individuals, families and communities to access, understand, appraise and apply health information in order to make judgements and take decisions in everyday life concerning health care, disease prevention and health promotion in order to maintain or improve their quality of life. It is considered to be a social determinant of health, and one of the key pillars in health promotion. Low health literacy is associated with poorer health, more illness and health inequalities, and it may make health systems less cost-effective. Evidence from the 2011 health literacy survey indicated that almost half of the adult population in eight Member States of the European Union had suboptimal general health literacy. Responses have included initiation of health literacy networks, policies, programmes and interventions at the regional, national and organizational levels. These initiatives require monitoring using frameworks and indicator sets that produce consistent and comparable population data and evaluation to determine the effectiveness of the policies and interventions.

The synthesis question

The objective of this report is to answer the question: "What is the evidence on the methods, frameworks and indicators used to evaluate health literacy policies, programmes and interventions at the regional, national and organizational levels?"

Types of evidence

This report used a scoping review to identify relevant documents in peer-reviewed and grey literature published between January 2013 and December 2018 in English, French, German, Russian and Spanish. To maximize the evidence identified, the search covered worldwide literature and experts in the field were also consulted.

Results

Of the 81 studies identified, 24 reported on an evaluation of a programme or intervention, and 57 used experimental research designs to report on the effect of an intervention on health literacy. The review found no evidence of the use of national or international datasets to evaluate policies, programmes or interventions, and no evidence on international, national or subnational health literacy evaluation frameworks. Studies were predominantly conducted in health service and education settings, and most measured health literacy at the personal/individual level using study-level data sources.

Studies that assessed the effect of an intervention on personal health literacy generally used quantitative methods based on previously published health literacy instruments or custom surveys/questionnaires containing questions on the outcomes of interest, for example changes in knowledge, behaviours or skills.

Qualitative and mixed-methods approaches, including surveys, semistructured interviews and focus groups, were used to evaluate health literacy programmes and interventions. In almost all of the mixed-methods studies, qualitative methods were used to inform a process evaluation of a programme or intervention, for example, participant satisfaction with a programme or intervention (acceptability); perceived benefits, strengths and limitations; facilitators and barriers to implementation; and programme sustainability. Four studies also reported an economic or financial analysis as part of the overall evaluation of a programme or intervention.

A wide range of health literacy measurement domains was identified. This included broad domains such as health literacy competencies and health literacy capacities, and more specific domains such as numeracy, comprehension, functional health literacy, interactive health literacy and critical health literacy. Other domains included understanding and awareness; changes in knowledge; changes in attitudes and beliefs; changes in skills, behaviours and practices; increased confidence and motivation; increased self-efficacy; and increased empowerment and decision-making.

Domains relating to an individual's interaction with health providers and services included adherence to medication, changes in help-seeking intentions and behaviours, changes in access to services, engagement with health providers (including communication) and trust in health providers.

Domains relating to organizational health literacy (responsiveness) included changes in the confidence, behaviours and health literacy practices of health practitioners; increased knowledge and awareness of health providers; increased understanding of health literacy concepts and practices; improved communication of health practitioners; increased health literacy competencies of teachers/staff; and increased health literacy responsiveness of schools.

Evaluation of health literacy programmes and interventions often involved multisectoral partnerships, the most common of which were academia–school partnerships, academia–community partnerships and academia–health service partnerships. Partnerships between academic institutions and government departments or bodies were also reported, while a small number of studies involved corporate or private sector partnerships. The roles and responsibilities of the personnel involved in these studies were generally not described, though some studies did report a joint responsibility for data collection, for example in academia–school or academia–health service partnerships in which teachers and clinicians, respectively, led the data collection while the academic researchers undertook data analysis.

The facilitators and barriers evaluated were broadly related to the following themes: skills and capacity of personnel, partnerships, time and budget constraints, and data collection methods and design. Other key facilitators identified through this review were the use of conceptual health literacy frameworks to guide programme evaluation, the development of evaluation guides including step-by-step instructions and standardized evaluation tools, clarity around roles and responsibilities in evaluation activities, appropriate allocation of resources, continuous monitoring to enable the early identification of areas for improvement, and government funding to support the evaluation of national programmes.

The level of resourcing (financial and human resources) required to evaluate policies, programmes and interventions was not specified in the studies identified for this report, but two studies suggested that the level of investment should match the scale and complexity of the programme and should be considered as part of the initial programme planning and design. There was little information on the scalability of the measures and tools used, with most relating to local settings such as clinics or a community.

Policy considerations

Based on the findings of this scoping review, the following policy considerations are proposed to strengthen the evaluation and monitoring of health literacy policies and programmes across Member States of the WHO European Region:

- develop indicator sets covering a broad range of health literacy domains that would be effective at both the subnational and national levels, facilitate measurement of population health literacy levels and provide data that could be compared across the Region;
- create measurement tools that are suitable for use across multiple settings and at multiple levels in order to support consistent data gathering on population health literacy in the Region;

- expand the use of qualitative and mixed-methods approaches for evaluating policies, programmes and interventions to enable an in-depth understanding of health literacy capacity and the cultural and contextual factors that influence it;
- increase the engagement of citizens, particularly vulnerable and marginalized communities and other relevant stakeholders, in participatory methods to develop measures of health literacy that are culturally and contextually relevant;
- expand the evaluation of health literacy at the organizational and system levels, including on governance, coordination and partnerships and the contextual factors contributing to health literacy; and
- establish partnerships for monitoring and evaluating health literacy policies and programmes, including with research institutions and organizations involved in the advancement of health literacy research, policy and practice.

1. INTRODUCTION

1.1 Background

1.1.1 Defining health literacy

In 2013, the WHO Regional Office for Europe published the report *Health literacy: the solid facts*, which identified health literacy as a stronger predictor of an individual's health status than income, employment status, education level and racial or ethnic group (1). Health literacy also follows a social gradient and can reinforce existing health inequalities; it may also make health systems less cost-effective. The report used the integrated, comprehensive definition of personal health literacy developed in the European Health Literacy Project (2009–2012) (2), which resulted in the European Health Literacy Survey (HLS-EU):

> Health literacy is linked to literacy and entails people's knowledge, motivation and competences to access, understand, appraise and apply health information in order to make judgements and take decisions in everyday life concerning health care, disease prevention and health promotion to maintain or improve quality of life during the life course.

Health literacy: the solid facts outlined a whole-of-society, multisectoral approach that addressed health literacy across the whole life-course and included community, educational and workplace settings; the continuum of health-care settings; and the range of potential methods of communication (e.g. oral, print, traditional media, social media and mobile health platforms). The report, furthermore, promoted the concept of the health-literate setting: "Health-literate settings infuse awareness of and action to strengthen health literacy throughout the policies, procedures and practices of the settings. They embrace strengthening health literacy as part of their core business" (1).

1.1.2 Health literacy in the WHO European Region

The 53 Member States of the WHO European Region have a combined population of 894 million but are diverse in their health, social, cultural and economic systems. Four are classified as having economies that are lower–middle income, five as upper–middle and 44 as high income (3).

The 2011 HLS-EU found that 47.6% of the adult population in the eight participating Member States (Austria, Bulgaria, Germany (North Rhine-Westphalia), Greece,

Ireland, the Netherlands, Poland and Spain) had suboptimal general health literacy (inadequate or problematic), and that this was linked to lower self-rated health, higher rates of chronic (i.e. long-term) health conditions, more adverse lifestyle choices (exercise, body mass index and alcohol) and higher use of health services (4).

This population evidence combined with an increased understanding of the relationship between health literacy and health outcomes has placed health literacy higher on the public policy agenda. At global level, the WHO *Shanghai Declaration on promoting health in the 2030 Agenda for Sustainable Development* (5) declared that health literacy is a critical determinant of health. This Declaration has provided a clear global mandate for governments to prioritize health literacy within public policies and has made it a global movement (6).

Health literacy has been on the agenda for almost two decades within the WHO European Region, resulting in widespread research activities, networks and implementation of health literacy projects. To manifest and measure health literacy in Europe, the European Commission supported the European Health Literacy Project (2009–2012), which was designed and executed by European stakeholders from eight European countries (2). The project generated a new, more detailed approach including a comprehensive definition, conceptual model and measurement instrument, plus a comparative survey. The project stimulated a wide range of activities at the local and national levels as well as European collaborations and conferences. The survey stimulated the measurement of population health literacy in other countries in the WHO European Region (Belgium, Czechia, Denmark, Germany, Hungary, Italy, Malta, Portugal and Switzerland). Reflecting the global, interconnected nature of the health literacy movement, the HLS-EU methodology has been used in surveys in numerous other countries in the WHO Europe Region and beyond, including Indonesia, Israel, Japan, Kazakhstan, Malaysia and Myanmar (7).

The Member States of the WHO European Region are committed to improving the information that underpins health policies. This is being undertaken as part of the WHO European Health Information Initiative (8). In 2018, a new WHO Action Network on Population and Organizational Health Literacy (M-POHL Network) was established, which aims to build an international version of the HLS-EU for monitoring (9) and an action network to support the use of health literacy for prevention and control of noncommunicable diseases was established in 2019. The WHO Regional Office for Europe in 2018 commissioned a report in the Health Evidence Network (HEN) synthesis series (report 57) to identify and synthesize evidence on health literacy policies and linked activities in the Region (10). The report identified 46 existing or developing policies from 19 of the 53 Member States. It found emerging evidence of successful activities at the individual and community levels, particularly in the societal areas of health and education, but it highlighted the lack of evidence of activities or their effectiveness at organizational or system level. Based on the evidence, HEN report 57 proposed strengthening the evidence base for health literacy, particularly in those societal areas with currently little or no published activity. It highlighted the importance of robust qualitative and quantitative measurement and evaluation of health literacy policies and interventions. It also emphasized the need to identify suitable evaluation frameworks and indicators for measuring health literacy policies and programmes across Member States in order to generate regular, high-quality and internationally comparable data and evidence on health literacy, and it stressed the potential benefits to be gained from sharing skills, resources and mutual learning across the Region.

1.1.3 Conceptual approaches to health literacy

Health literacy is understood as a relational, interactive or contextual concept. Accordingly, a basic distinction is the health literacy of individuals or populations (here we refer to it as personal health literacy). Community health literacy in this report refers to studies that measured individual/personal health literacy of a specific population or target group. Organizational health literacy encompasses the professional and organizational characteristics that enable professionals, organizations or systems to be responsive to people's needs and to ameliorate health literacy barriers.

Personal health literacy

There are multiple, and to some degree overlapping, definitions of personal health literacy. In 2012, Sørensen et al. identified 17 definitions of health literacy and 12 conceptual models (11), and more are emerging as the science develops. Conceptual definitions vary in their dimensions (e.g. finding, understanding, appraising, interacting and acting on information for health in various roles and societal settings). Generic models define antecedents or determinants (the factors underlying health or causing literacy) and identify the consequences of health literacy and health literacy activities (e.g. lifestyles or health behaviours, indicators of health status, and use and outcomes of health-care services and related costs). The health literacy definition and model chosen for a health literacy policy and its related activities are key to measurement and evaluation. The choice will be driven by the context and setting; it will determine the key actors and likely consequences, and it should lead towards the choice of the optimal measurement tools to capture evidence of those consequences. A detailed examination of health literacy definitions and frameworks is not within the scope of this report; however, some key examples are given here to illustrate the above points. One important distinction within personal health literacy is between a clinical and public health perspective.

Clinical (or medical) perspectives. Here, there is a focus on the literacy, language and numeracy skills required by individuals as users to perform tasks within a health-care environment. This also has an organizational health literacy aspect in that it implies that organizations and practitioners should have skills to identify and address barriers to providing care for patients with a range of different health literacy capacities and needs (12,13). Measurement and evaluation activities with this clinical perspective will usually take place in medical settings and may include only specific medical conditions. Outcomes focus on the capacity of patients to comply with medical advice and treatment and their ability to self-manage their medical conditions.

Public health perspectives. In this view, health literacy is an asset for healthy living that can be built through community empowerment, civic engagement and social action; it is also a determinant of positive health and well-being (14,15). Public health literacy activities can take place in a wide variety of settings and in the context of peoples' everyday lives. Outcomes include the capacity to understand information for health and also the capacity to evaluate and make decisions for individual and collective action (16).

As a consequence of the trend to use a more comprehensive understanding of the terms health and literacy, definitions and measures for specific aspects of personal health literacy have evolved to encompass specific sections of the population (e.g. different age groups or different lifestyles), specific aspects of health (e.g. condition or topic) and specific types of communication (e.g. oral, written or digital) (4). Two examples of this are given.

Digital health literacy. This concept is attracting increasing attention because means of communication are changing rapidly through advances in digital technology (e.g. extending from oral or written methods). Electronic/Internet sources are now an important method for finding information to make judgements and take decisions (for health) in everyday life (11). A widely used definition states that digital health literacy is "the ability to seek, find, understand, and appraise health information from electronic sources and apply the knowledge gained to addressing or solving a health problem" (17).

Mental health literacy. The concept of mental health literacy developed separately from the wider health literacy field. Early definitions focused on peoples' knowledge, attitudes and beliefs about mental disorders that aid their recognition, management or prevention (18). Recently, the definition has evolved to include capacities to obtain and maintain mental health and to seek mental health help when needed (19). The outcomes of mental health literacy activities, and hence the indicators of change studied and the tools used to demonstrate that change, may, consequently, vary widely according to the definition of mental health literacy around which the study centres.

Organizational health literacy

Organizational health literacy models and frameworks focus on the relationship between the health literacy skills of individuals and the complexity of health services and systems (20,21). It refers to the skills and responsiveness of organizations and practitioners to identify and address barriers to providing care for patients with a range of different health literacy capacities and needs (12,13). Domains focus on aspects of leadership and organizational principles, culture, systems and processes. There is some variation in the terminology applied within the field (22); however, there are already a number of reviews that provide conceptual and operational guidance for this rapidly evolving field of research, practice and policy (22–27). The most comprehensive concepts and frameworks have been developed in Australia (28,29), Europe (27,30) and the United States of America (24,31).

1.1.4 Objectives of this report

HEN report 57 highlighted existing health literacy policies and interventions in the WHO European Region and outlined a limited number of evaluation studies measuring the implementation of health literacy policies (10). One of the key policy considerations suggested in that report was to undertake qualitative and quantitative evaluations of health literacy policies, programmes and interventions. This is particularly pertinent considering that governments are increasingly developing national health literacy policies.

This report aims to improve understanding of these gaps with a scoping review of the best available evidence to address the following synthesis question: "What is the evidence on the methods, frameworks and indicators used to evaluate health literacy policies, programmes and interventions at the regional, national and organizational levels?"

1.2 Methodology

A scoping review was undertaken to identify the best available evidence on the methods, frameworks and indicators used to evaluate health literacy policies, programmes and interventions published between 1 January 2013 and 31 December 2018. As the science of evaluating health literacy policies and programmes is relatively new, it was likely that the available evidence specific to any one region would be limited. Consequently, a global search was used to find the best available evidence that could be applied to the WHO European Region. A search was carried out of peer-reviewed publications in English, French, German, Russian and Spanish and of the grey literature using the Google search engine in English only. Relevant documents were also sourced from the HEN report 57, which identified evidence on health literacy policies (and linked activities) across the WHO European Region (10); the Health Literacy Toolshed[1] (32); and by enquiries with international experts. Documents had to include the term health literacy (or equivalent translated terms).

A total of 2312 peer-reviewed articles were found after removal of duplicates. Full text screening resulted in 68 articles, to which were added five from the grey literature search, two from expert consultation and six from report 57. The 81 identified studies included 24 reporting on an evaluation of a programme or intervention (i.e. implementation, acceptability or appropriateness) (33–56) and 57 reporting measurement of the effect of an intervention on health literacy (i.e. did not include an assessment of the intervention or programme itself) (19,57–112).

Annex 1 has full details of the search strategy and inclusion criteria.

1. Health Literacy Toolshed is a curated web-based repository of tools that measure one or more dimension of health literacy at the personal level. Tools included must have at least one validation study published in the peer-reviewed literature that meets reporting standards for a minimum set of validation characteristics. Inclusion of a tool in the Toolshed is not a blanket endorsement. At the time of writing, there are 191 tools listed.

2. RESULTS

Of the 81 studies identified in the review, 24 reported on an evaluation of a programme or intervention (33–56) and 57 reported on the effect of an intervention on health literacy, using experimental designs such as randomized controlled trials, community-based cluster trials, brief clinical health service interventions or other research-oriented study designs (19,57–112). The results of the review are outlined in the following sections:

- 2.1: general features of the studies;
- 2.2: evaluation frameworks and logic models;
- 2.3: methods (quantitative, qualitative, mixed methods, economic evaluation, health literacy measurement instruments, and sources for data and collection frequency);
- 2.4: measurement domains and indicators;
- 2.5: partnerships and coordination for health literacy measurement;
- 2.6: facilitators and barriers to health literacy measurement;
- 2.7: resources and scalability; and
- 2.8: evaluation of health literacy in the WHO European Region.

Case studies illustrate approaches to health literacy measurement undertaken in the WHO European Region.

2.1 General features of the studies

As might be expected from an emerging and evolving area of policy and practice, this report did not identify any published evaluation of national or subnational health literacy policies and identified only a small number of evaluations of national programmes. Some of the studies identified took place in more than one setting and/or at more than one societal level. One issue is that health literacy definitions and frameworks vary widely in both what they encompass and what terms they use. Addressing this issue is not within the scope of this report but an overview of relevant concepts is given in Annex 2.

2.1.1 Levels of measurement

The majority of studies ($n = 67$) were conducted at local level with measurements at a single site or at multiple sites in a single city or town. Four studies were conducted at subnational level across multiple cities/towns but within a single state, territory or county (33,57–59). Nine studies were conducted at national level, which included evaluations of national government programmes or of research projects implemented on a national scale across multiple states, territories or counties (34–38,60–63). Only one study was conducted at international level and this measured the impact of an online intervention across various countries (64).

2.1.2 Settings

The studies were conducted predominantly in health service settings (n = 44) and education settings (including schools, universities and adult learning centres; n = 43), with a small number conducted across workplace (n = 8), community (the lived environment; n = 18) and digital/media settings (n = 10). There were 33 studies that involved implementation and measurement of health literacy across two or more of these settings.

2.1.3 Societal level

Almost all of the studies in this report (n = 79) focused on health literacy at individual level. Eight studies focused on community health literacy (community in this report refers to studies that measure personal health literacy of those in a specific population or target group) (35,36,39–42,65,66). Five studies focused on health literacy at organizational level (33,36,43,44,67), for example improvements to the organizational environment or improvements to the skills of the health workforce. There was only one study focused on health literacy at system/legislative level (38); this evaluated a national health literacy partnership to determine the functions and effectiveness of the partnership in governing the implementation and monitoring of national health literacy goals.

2.1.4 Health literacy topics

A large number of studies addressed and measured personal health literacy in general (n = 30) and mental health literacy (n = 28), including specific mental health conditions. In addition, a number of studies addressed and measured condition- or topic-specific health literacy, including literacy in digital health (n = 5) chronic disease (and risk factors; n = 6), nutrition (n = 2), diabetes (n = 3), smoking advertising and promotion (n = 1), cancer (n = 1), medication (n = 4), sexual health (n = 2), climate change/environmental health (n = 3), eye health (n = 1), oral health (n = 2) and malaria (n = 1).

2.2 Evaluation frameworks and logic models

There were no international, national or subnational health literacy evaluation frameworks identified through this review, and evidence on the use of evaluation frameworks was limited. There were some studies that utilized well-known health literacy conceptual models or frameworks to inform research project or programme evaluation (11,16,45). Three studies developed programme logic models or theory of change frameworks to guide their implementation and evaluation (35,43,44).

2.2.1 Health literacy conceptual models or frameworks

The integrated model of health literacy of Sørensen et al. (11) combined clinical and public health perspectives of health literacy. It conceptualized health literacy as a process of empowerment and emphasized the influence of social and situational determinants on health literacy. It also reinforced the concept of health literacy as the knowledge and skill set required across a continuum, from health care (individual level) through to disease prevention and health promotion (population level), which requires action outside of health-care settings. This framework contains three health action/continuum domains: (i) health care, (ii) disease prevention, and (iii) health promotion. There are four types of competency (capability domains): (i) access/obtain information relevant to health, (ii) understand information relevant to health, (iii) process/appraise information relevant to health to decide what is relevant, and (iv) apply information relevant to health to communicate and make decisions to maintain and improve health. The combination of these two sets creates a matrix of 12 domains. The model also describes a range of health literacy-related outcomes, including health service use, health costs, health behaviours, health outcomes, participation, empowerment, equity and sustainability.

Nutbeam's asset model conceptualized health literacy as an asset for personal empowerment and broader social change (16). The model described three levels or domains of health literacy: (i) functional health literacy, which relates to the reading and writing skills required to function effectively in everyday situations; (ii) interactive health literacy, which encompasses the advanced cognitive and literacy skills as well as the social skills required to actively participate in everyday activities; and (iii) critical health literacy, which encompasses the advanced cognitive skills and social skills required to critically analyse information and to use this information to exert greater control over life events and situations. Interactive health literacy would include extracting health information, deriving meaning from different forms of communication and applying this information under various and changing circumstances.

The environmental health literacy framework describes three dimensions of environmental health literacy: (i) awareness and knowledge, (ii) skills and self-efficacy, and (iii) community change (actions) (45). It was used to assess four communities in Arizona, United States, with known environmental health stressors (45).

2.2.2 Evaluation informed by logic or theory of change models

There were three studies that developed programme logic models or theory of change frameworks to guide their implementation and evaluation, including one on a national programme in the United Kingdom (35) and two on local projects in Australia (43,44). Logic models and theories of change support the evaluation of programme implementation and outcomes by describing the links and assumptions between the programme inputs (i.e. financial and human resources) and activities and the intended outputs (i.e. products or deliverables) and outcomes in the short, medium and long terms. Each framework described outcomes at the individual and organizational or system levels.

The Skilled for Health Programme in the United Kingdom used a theory of change framework to derive individual and organizational outcomes (35). The outcomes for individuals were increased life skills, increased confidence, increased interest in health, better job opportunities, healthier living and improved health. The outcomes for organizations were reduced sickness-related absence from the workplace and increased uptake of education programmes.

A logic model was used in a randomized controlled trial to describe a community-based preventive health intervention in Australia (43). The individual outcomes were improved knowledge and understanding, improved health literacy and improved health outcomes. It also described outcomes for health-care providers, including improved risk factor assessments for patients, increased understanding of the impact of health literacy on patients, increased skills to address health literacy of patients and improved risk factor management of patients. Organizational or system level outcomes were better systems for recording and monitoring patients.

Health attitudes and behaviours formed during childhood greatly influence adult health patterns, and one Australian programme examined a school-based health literacy programme (44). A logic model was used to describe outcomes that were mainly at organizational or system level. These included developing a health literacy action plan; embedding health literacy in the curriculum; improving health literacy leadership, competencies and partnerships; decreasing literacy-related barriers for vulnerable groups; making better use of health literacy resources; and creating sustainable health literacy-responsive schools. It also described outcomes relating to school stakeholders, including students and staff: greater awareness of health literacy, improved health literacy (skills, knowledge and practices) and improved health outcomes.

2.3 Methods

2.3.1 Quantitative methods

A large number of studies in this report used only quantitative methods to measure health literacy (19,57–60,62–103). These studies predominantly assessed the effect of an intervention on health literacy. Almost all of the quantitative studies involved the use of surveys or questionnaires as the method of data collection, many of which were self-administered or interviewer administered/assisted using paper-based surveys, although a small number were self-administered using Internet-based surveys.

Quantitative studies frequently used previously published health literacy instruments to measure health literacy, including test-based and self-report measures (sections 2.3.5 and 2.3.6), or in some instances a smaller subset of questions from these instruments. There were also a number of studies that developed customized surveys or questionnaires. In these, the questions were developed by the authors to measure individual outcomes of interest (e.g. changes in knowledge, behaviours or skills) or to evaluate programme implementation and outcomes (58,59,65,66,69,71,83–85,94,95,97,101,104).

There were a small number of studies that combined the use of a health literacy survey or questionnaire with clinical measures (e.g. body mass index) (82), observation checklists (104) or knowledge checklists (85).

2.3.2 Qualitative methods

Only four studies used a purely qualitative methodology and these were all studies involving an evaluation: two small-scale health education programmes in the United States (46) and Australia (47), a national health education programme in Sweden (34) and a national health literacy partnership/alliance in Austria (38).

In-depth, semistructured interviews were used to evaluate the impact of a cancer survivorship programme in the United States on the health literacy of adolescents and young adults and on communication between survivors and health-care providers (46). Interviews were conducted with four stakeholder groups: cancer survivors, health-care providers, hospital administrators and advocates for cancer survivors. In addition to evaluating the impact of the programme on health literacy and communication, the interviews explored participant perceptions about opportunities to sustain the programme, what they valued about it, what elements were most important and what were the barriers to participating in education programmes. The interviews were conducted with a small sample of participants and were guided by an interview format tailored to each group.

One Australian study used focus groups to evaluate a small community-based health literacy programme to determine how the design, approach and delivery mode resulted in increased health literacy and behaviour change for participants (47). A total of 22 people participated in four focus groups, which represented nearly half of all programme participants. The focus groups were guided by a semistructured interview format and analysed according to four themes including autonomy and competence and relatedness (components of self-determination theory) and a separate but related theme of empowerment.

A study on a national sexual health literacy programme for newly arrived migrants in Sweden used in-depth, semistructured interviews to explore the perceptions of female participants about the content and delivery of the programme and whether it had enhanced their sexual health as well as their understanding and capacities in relation to sexual health (34). Purposive sampling was used to engage female refugees from the three largest language groups at the time: Arabic, Dari and Somali. Nine women were interviewed for the study out of the 19 who were eligible in that block of education sessions. An interview guide containing four broad topics was developed for the interviews. The first topic explored participants' experiences of receiving sexual health information in the context of life circumstances, culture and previous experiences. The other three topics covered the domains of Nutbeam's health literacy model (functional, interactive, critical), including participants' perceptions of sexual health knowledge and attitudes, motivation and reflections.

An evaluation of the Austrian Platform for Health Literacy (ÖPGK) (38) (Case study 1) used a combination of key informant interviews, document reviews and analysis and observations at meetings and partnership events to evaluate the structures, functions and governance of the partnership, and identify areas for its improvement.

Case study 1. Partnership evaluation of ÖPGK

ÖPGK was established by the Federal Health Commission (Bundesgesundheitskommission) as a governance mechanism for supporting the implementation of one of Austria's 10 national health goals: strengthening the health literacy of the population. ÖPGK consists of a coordination office and core team of experts, including from implementing organizations and federal ministries.

An external evaluation of the partnership examined the extent to which the ÖPGK structures and functions had been established as intended, and whether the ÖPGK was working effectively, including progress made towards achieving its goals and targets (38).

The evaluation involved multiple qualitative methods and participation by a range of stakeholder groups involved in the platform. First, a document review and analysis was carried out for strategy papers and reports, meeting documents and annual reports, conferences, and the website. Secondly, in-depth, semistructured interviews were undertaken with 17 participants, including representatives of the core team (includes technical experts and operational staff), the coordination office, the Federal Ministry of Health and Women's Affairs, the ÖPGK membership and the Board of Trustees of the primary funding body (Fund Healthy Austria). Finally, participant observations were undertaken at ÖPGK meetings and conferences.

Together, these were used to identify key strengths and limitations of the partnership in achieving its functions and goals, its key successes, and recommendations for improving the platform in the future.

2.3.3 Mixed methods

A mixed-methods approach was used in 30 studies (33,35–37,39–45,48–56,61,104–112), 20 of which involved an evaluation of a programme or intervention (33,35–37, 39–45,48–56). The most common mixed-methods study design was the use of a quantitative survey in combination with semistructured interviews (33,35, 39–43,46,49,50,54–56,61,107). The quantitative component was generally used to complete a formal assessment of health literacy using either a published health literacy instrument (see sections 2.3.5 and 2.3.6) or a custom survey developed specifically to address the objectives of the study. The interviews were usually conducted with a sample of study participants, but some studies also involved other stakeholders with an interest or role in the intervention or programme (e.g. health professionals, trainers). Five studies used quantitative surveys together with focus groups (44,47,52,53,106) and three studies combined quantitative surveys, interviews and focus groups (36,48,51).

In almost all of the mixed-methods studies, the interviews and focus groups were used to inform a process evaluation of the programme or intervention. This included, for example, an assessment of participant satisfaction with a programme or intervention (acceptability); the perceived benefits, strengths and limitations; facilitators and barriers to implementation; and programme sustainability (see section 2.4.3 for details). However, there was one study that used in-depth interviews to explore the critical health literacy skills of participants (48), and another that used Photovoice to explore participants' health literacy-related experiences, strengths and suggestions for system improvements (40) (Case study 2).

Case study 2. Using Photovoice in the evaluation of a health literacy programme

Photovoice is a qualitative, participatory method using a combination of photographs to highlight themes or issues. It is used to engage and empower marginalized population groups, as well as culturally and linguistically diverse communities (113). A programme targeting south Asian young men with diabetes in Stoke-on-Trent, United Kingdom, used Photovoice to explore participants' health literacy-related experiences, strengths and suggestions for system improvements as part of an evaluation of a local health literacy programme (40). Photovoice was used to enable participants to explore and express their experiences of navigating the health-care system, identify their personal health literacy-related strengths, identify the system changes that needed to occur to support them to manage their condition and to inform/educate policy- and decision-makers about the participants' realities and experiences of living with the condition.

A small number of studies combined quantitative with qualitative open-ended survey questions (37,45,104,108,109). In these studies, the qualitative survey was used either to supplement a quantitative assessment of health literacy (i.e. through open-ended questions) or to assess participants' experiences and satisfaction as part of a process evaluation of an intervention or programme. In one study of digital health literacy, an open-ended survey was used to explore and assess health literacy skills qualitatively (108).

Other qualitative methods used as part of a mixed-methods approach included observations (use of notes and journals by participants and researchers) (40,105), document reviews (audits of meeting minutes and project documents) (39–41,112), case studies (35), learning network events and workshops (33,44) and feedback sessions (111). Again, these methods were generally used to inform a process evaluation of programmes and interventions.

Other quantitative methods used as part of a mixed-methods approach included an organizational self-assessment checklist, which was used to detect changes in the health literacy responsiveness of schools before and after a whole-of-school programme (section 2.3.6) (44), and a self-assessment tool, which was used to report changes in health behaviours and learning outcomes (35).

2.3.4 Economic evaluation methods

Four studies reported using a form of economic or financial analysis as part of an overall evaluation of a programme or intervention. A study on a school-based education programme in the United Kingdom carried out a cost–benefit analysis by estimating the cost per unit change in health and nutrition literacy outcomes, based on changes in scores before and after implementation (105). An evaluation of a large national programme in Germany (With Migrants for Migrants – Intercultural Health in Germany (MiMi)) is undertaken annually and incorporates a cost–effectiveness assessment using quantitative and qualitative methods to determine the efficiency and effectiveness of the programme; however, the specific details of how this analysis is undertaken were not provided (36).

A chronic disease prevention programme in Australia evaluated the impacts and outcomes of a mobile health-enhanced preventive intervention in primary care and assessed changes in health literacy, behavioural outcomes and clinical outcomes (43). The study protocol incorporated an economic evaluation to determine the overall cost of establishing and implementing the intervention, and to estimate the costs of clinical service delivery compared with the costs of referral into and uptake of community-based programmes (43). The costs were assessed using linked data from public medical insurance and hospital data.

A cost–effectiveness analysis was undertaken in a Chinese study on a digital intervention to improve health literacy using text messaging of health education information (99). In this study, cost–effectiveness was calculated as a ratio of the cost of sending the messages divided by the effectiveness of the intervention on health literacy, which was measured using the Test of Functional Health Literacy in Adults (114).

2.3.5 Health literacy measurement instruments: personal health literacy

There is a long tradition of measuring personal or population health literacy and a tendency of internal differentiation into different aspects of personal health literacy (e.g. mental health literacy). In contrast, there are fewer studies of organizational health literacy (responsiveness) or health-literate (health-care) organizations (section 2.3.6).

In the studies included in this report, 58 measurement tools were used to measure personal health literacy, including 31 published health literacy instruments (Annex 3 lists their characteristics) and 27 custom (study-specific) tools. Many of the published instruments used in the studies measure personal health literacy in general (40,41,47–49,52,53,55,67,76,77,79,81,82,96,99,100,102,103,107,108); some measure individuals' mental health literacy (19,37,50,51,57,62,64,68,70,72,73,78,88–93,109,111) and a small number measure other condition- or topic-specific types of health literacy, including digital health (43,53,74,76,77,108), nutrition (105), diabetes (52), smoking advertising and promotion (75,98), malaria (87) and high blood pressure (80). Health literacy instruments were often used in research studies to measure the effect of an intervention on health literacy. Some of these tools were also used to measure health literacy in the evaluation studies in this report and are discussed in more detail here.

The general health literacy instruments used as part of evaluation studies were the All Aspects of Health Literacy Scale (AAHLS) (115), Short Test of Functional Health Literacy in Adults (STOFHLA) (40,116), Health Literacy Questionnaire (HLQ) (41,43,54,55,117), e-Health Literacy Scale (e-HEALS) (43,53,118), HLS-EU (49,119), Ishikawa Health Literacy Survey (120) and the Single Item Literacy Screener (SILS) (55,121). The instruments used in mental health literacy evaluation studies were the Anxiety Literacy Scale (51,122), Depression Literacy Scale (51,123), Mental Health Literacy Scale (51,124) and Mental Health Knowledge Schedule (50,125,126).

The Depression Literacy Scale, Anxiety Literacy Scale and STOFHLA are all test-based (objective) measures. STOFHLA was used as part of a multimethod evaluation of a local health literacy programme targeting south Asian young men with diabetes in Stoke-on-Trent, United Kingdom (40). It assesses numeracy, reading and comprehension and uses categorical scoring to assess individuals as having inadequate, marginal or adequate health literacy (scoring range, 0–100) (116). Both the Anxiety Literacy Scale and the Depression Literacy Scale assess mental health knowledge/awareness/attitudes using a true/false questionnaire in which each correct answer scores one point and the overall score (range, 0–22) is used to determine high or low knowledge, awareness and attitudes in relation to depression and anxiety (122,123,127,128). Both Scales were used together with the Mental Health Literacy Scale to evaluate the impact of a multistrategy, community sports-based programme that aimed to improve the mental health literacy of adolescent males and their parents (51). The Mental Health Literacy Scale contains test-based and self-report measures across six domains: (i) ability to recognize disorders, (ii) knowledge of where to seek information, (iii) knowledge of risk factors and causes, (iv) knowledge of self-treatment, (v) knowledge of professional help available, and (vi) attitudes that promote recognition or appropriate help-seeking behaviour (124).

The AAHLS, e-HEALS, HLQ, HLS-EU and Ishikawa Health Literacy Survey are self-report (subjective) instruments that measure health literacy based on people's own perceptions of their capabilities within the settings in which they live. The AAHLS was used as part of a mixed-method evaluation of a community family learning programme in the United Kingdom, which had a particular emphasis on its impact on critical health literacy (48). The AAHLS contains 14 questions to assess health literacy skills across four domains/scales: (i) functional, (ii) interactive, (iii) critical, and (iv) empowerment (115). Questions in the first three domains have three response options: often, sometimes and rarely. Health literacy is measured as a summary score and has the ability to show specific health literacy strengths and limitations across the four domains.

The HLQ was used in four mixed-methods evaluations, all conducted in Australia (41,43,54,55). The HLQ is a self-administered questionnaire containing 44 questions to assess health literacy across nine domains/scales: (i) feeling understood and supported by health-care providers, (ii) having sufficient information to manage my health, (iii) actively managing my health, (iv) having social support for health, (v) appraising health information, (vi) having the ability to actively engage with health-care providers, (vii) navigating the health-care system, (viii) having the ability to find good health information, and (ix) understanding health information well enough to know what to do (117). It also contains nine demographic questions, including age, sex, country of birth and whether people speak English at home (117). Each scale is measured independently to show specific health literacy strengths and limitations. There are four response options for the first five scales (strongly disagree, disagree, agree, strongly agree) and five for the last four scales (cannot do or always difficult, usually difficult, sometimes difficult, usually easy, always easy) with a score of 1–4 or 1–5.

In one Australian study, the HLQ was used in combination with e-HEALS to allow a more comprehensive assessment of both general health literacy and digital health literacy skills (43). The e-HEALS questionnaire assesses digital health literacy skills specifically relating to online/Internet-based health information. It is a computer-administered survey containing eight questions relating to knowledge, skills and confidence to navigate and find information on the Internet (118). A community library programme in the United States also used e-HEALS to evaluate the impact of a consumer health workshop (53).

Another Australian study combined the use of the HLQ with the SILS (55). The SILS is a single item screener that is used to rapidly assess inadequate health literacy in terms of ability to use printed health material. It specifically asks, "How often do you need to have someone help you when you read instructions, pamphlets, or other written material from your doctor or pharmacy" (121), with five response options (never, rarely, sometimes, often, always) scoring 1–5. A score of more than 2 on this scale is considered to reflect difficulty in reading printed health-related material.

The HLS-EU questionnaire was used as part of a mixed-methods evaluation of the health literacy capacities developed through participating in a community-based cardiovascular programme in Ireland (48). HLS-EU contains 47 questions across three domains and 12 subscales. The three domains are health care, disease prevention and health promotion. For each domain there are four subscales: (i) access/obtain information, (ii) understand information relevant to health, (iii) process/appraise information relevant to health, and (iv) apply/use information relevant to health. The response options for each subscale are scored from 1 to 5 (very difficult, difficult, easy, very easy and don't know) (119). The results of all scales are combined to construct a category score of health literacy as insufficient, problematic, sufficient or excellent. In the study, the HLS-EU was administered for a quantitative assessment of health literacy levels, but it was also used to inform the development of an interview guide for qualitative exploration of health literacy capabilities (48).

An Australian study combined the use of the Ishikawa Health Literacy Survey with a study-specific survey to evaluate an adult education programme for socially disadvantaged adults (56). The study-specific survey assessed functional health literacy skills relating to the course content. The Ishikawa Health Literacy Survey was used to evaluate a broader range of health literacy skills. The survey was originally developed to assess the health literacy of patients with diabetes but is also used with patients with chronic disease. It contains 14 questions across three domains/ scales: functional, communicative (interactive) and critical (120). The response options for each scale are scored from 1 to 4 (never, rarely, sometimes, often) and are summed for each scale and divided by the number of questions in each scale to provide an overall health literacy score.

A study on the impact of a school-based programme on mental health literacy and stigma in the United Kingdom used the stigma-related Mental Health Knowledge Schedule to assess mental health knowledge and attitudes before and after the intervention (50). The Schedule contains 12 questions that assess stigma in relation to help-seeking, recognition, support, employment, treatment and recovery, as well as for knowledge of mental illness conditions. The response options for each question are scored from 1 to 5 (agree strongly, agree slightly, neither agree nor disagree, disagree slightly, disagree strongly), and the total score is calculated as the sum of all responses (125,126).

2.3.6 Health literacy measurement instruments: organizational health literacy

Measurement of organizational health literacy is a much more recent tradition compared with assessments of personal health literacy (27).

Two tools were identified that had been used to measure at least one aspect of organizational health literacy (health literacy responsiveness) as part of a programme or intervention. The first was an organizational self-assessment checklist (HeLLO Tas!) (129) used as part of a needs assessment to inform a whole-of-school health literacy action plan in Australia to improve the health literacy responsiveness of school environments (44). The HeLLO Tas! checklist consists of six domains: (i) involving consumers in planning and evaluation processes, (ii) supporting the workforce to use effective health literacy practices, (iii) meeting the needs of diverse communities, (iv) enabling access and navigation, (v) communicating, and (vi) having leadership and management (129). HeLLO Tas! was administered again at the completion of the programme to detect changes in health literacy awareness, competencies and responsiveness of the school environment. The checklist was completed using a teacher-led workshop format involving a small group of teachers.

The other organizational tool was a health literacy instrument designed to measure the communication skills of health professionals, including their written and oral skills as well as patient–provider collaboration (79). This tool was used in a randomized controlled trial to assess the impact of a communication training intervention on the skills of primary health-care providers (79).

2.3.7 Sources for data and collection frequency

No policies, programmes or interventions could be identified that were evaluated using international or national indicator sets. The Geneva Gay Men's Health Survey used population survey data routinely collected (every 4–5 years) at city level (68). The survey included questions on mental health literacy, including on depression, perceived risk and first-aid response; help-seeking beliefs about people and professionals; help-seeking beliefs about substances (including medications); and help-seeking beliefs about activities (including therapies).

All other studies identified for this report used study-specific data sources, which were collected as part of the study design using the tools and methods described in previous sections.

Some studies conducted within health services also used secondary data routinely collected at the study site, such as medical records (110) or clinical measures (43,82). These secondary sources were analysed in conjunction with health literacy assessments (using health literacy instruments) in order to show an association between changes in health literacy and other clinical outcomes as a result of an intervention.

A pre–post design was commonly used in which health literacy was measured at baseline and immediately following the intervention to assess its short-term impact on the health literacy outcomes of interest. Many of these involved a pre–post design in which there was a single follow-up survey at least one month and up to 12 months following the intervention, while some involved a repeat follow-up design in which there were at least two follow-up surveys after the intervention. The repeat surveys were generally conducted at six, 12 and 18 months following the intervention (43,44,54,80,85); however, some had shorter follow-up intervals (55,62,69,91,95), and one had a follow-up survey two years after the intervention (57). In most of the studies, the repeat designs used quantitative methods, but two studies also involved a repeat interview methodology (49,55).

2.4 Measurement domains and indicators

This section describes the domains used to measure health literacy in research and evaluation studies. The term domain was often used interchangeably with the terms indicators, measures and outcomes in the literature. The term domain is used in this section to describe the areas of measurement that are generally assessed using multiple indicators or questions.

While the review found that no international or national indicator sets had been used to evaluate policies, programmes or interventions, most studies reported on programme/intervention measurement domains and indicators, which are described here. It should be noted that, due to the concept having developed separately from the general health literacy field, mental health literacy indicators may reflect different domains to those in other health literacy studies.

2.4.1 Outcome domains for personal health literacy

Outcome domains and indicators are used to monitor and evaluate the intermediate effects of an intervention or programme on individuals or communities, for example effect on knowledge, attitudes, beliefs or behaviours (130).

A number of studies specified a broad indicator of health literacy, for example an increase in health literacy, health literacy competencies or health literacy capacities. This included studies that were specific to a topic, such as increased nutrition or diabetes literacy (41,43,48,49,52,75,76,81,82,87,96,98,100,101,103,107). Some studies were more specific about the aspect of health literacy being measured, for example changes in numeracy or comprehension or changes in functional, interactive and critical health literacy (40,42,55,56,102).

The health literacy studies identified in this report also frequently contained one or more of the following domains: increased understanding and awareness, changes in knowledge, and changes in attitudes and beliefs (34,35,39,42,45,55,60,61,75,77,98, 110). In addition to these, some studies also measured at least one of the following domains: changes in skills, behaviours and practices; increased confidence; increased motivation; increased self-efficacy; increased empowerment; and improved decision-making (34,39,40,43,45,47,55,56,60,65,74,76,79,80,84,86,94,107).

Some studies measured domains relating to an individual's interaction with health providers and services, including adherence to medication, changes in help-seeking intentions and behaviours, changes in access to services, engagement with health providers (including communication) and trust in health providers (35,40,42,43,72,74,79,84,105,107).

Only two studies reported on broader social change or action domains: one measured understanding of social determinants (49) and the other measured changes in perceptions of civic responsibility (106).

Digital health literacy. There were three studies that specified an outcome domain for digital health literacy, which in each was broadly stated as changes or increases in e-health literacy (43,74,76). While not specifically stated, use of the e-HEALS instrument suggests that the specific domains measured were likely to be knowledge, skills and confidence to navigate and find information on the Internet.

Mental health literacy. The domains described in the mental health literacy studies can be broadly grouped into three categories:

- domains focusing on an individual's own mental health, which included increased skills in relation to mental health (51,57,64,69,73,92,93); increased knowledge or understanding about mental health, including disorders, symptoms and treatment (19,37,57,62,69,73,78,85,89–91,95,109,111); changes in help-seeking attitudes, beliefs or intentions (37,50,62,68,73,78,85,93,109); and an individual's perceptions of the social support available (measured in one study) (85);
- domains focusing on supporting other people, which included increased confidence or intentions to support someone with a mental disorder (37,57,95,109,111) and increased knowledge about how to behave and act when with a person with a mental disorder (57); and
- domains focusing on individuals' attitudes towards mental health, with implications for improving broader social norms, where the two domains frequently used were changes in attitudes towards people with mental disorders (19,57,64,85,88–90,95,111) and decreased stigma about mental illness (37,50, 62,64,69,73,78,92,93,95,109).

2.4.2 Outcome domains for organizational health literacy

Studies that examined organizational health literacy included health service-based quality improvement activities, a general health literacy training course for health and social service professionals, health literacy training for medical or health students, and one programme that aimed to increase the health literacy responsiveness of school settings.

The studies on health service-based quality improvement activities contained domains on changes in the confidence, behaviours and health literacy practices of health providers/practitioners (54) and increased knowledge of health providers (59). A study on a general health literacy course for health and social service professionals measured increased understanding of health literacy concepts and practices, and intentions to adopt health literacy practices within their organization (33).

The studies that evaluated training courses for medical/health professionals all contained domains on their knowledge about health literacy (97,101,104,112) and attitudes about health literacy (i.e. its level of importance in patient outcomes) (97,101,104,112). Some also included domains on communication skills (101,104,112) and increased confidence to address the health literacy needs of patients (101,112).

The programme to promote the health literacy responsiveness of schools reported on three organizational level domains: increased health literacy awareness of teachers and staff, increased health literacy competencies of teachers and staff, and increased health literacy responsiveness of schools (44).

2.4.3 Process indicators

Process indicators are used in programme monitoring and evaluation in order to assess implementation progress, challenges and overall quality, as well as programme inputs, outputs and costs. They are also used to evaluate the extent to which a programme is implemented as planned; the strengths, limitations and benefits of a programme; and the elements of a programme that have resulted in change and improvements. Collecting data on process indicators allows programmers to make quality improvements during programme implementation, and to inform decisions about future programmes (130).

A number of process indicators were identified in the studies in this report. Some studies measured programme reach by collecting data on the number of participants involved in a programme or the number of professionals trained in a course (36,46,67,106). Reach was also reported in terms of success with engaging the target population (e.g. Roma people living in Ireland (39)). Other studies included output measures, such as the number of resources developed and distributed as part of a health education programme (46) and the number/type of relationships established between the target population and health service providers (39).

In a study protocol on an intervention that aimed to increase the knowledge and skills of obese and overweight people with low health literacy, the authors evaluated intervention fidelity by measuring the percentage of health professionals (physicians and practice nurses) who participated in training and the percentage of clients who received several elements of the intervention (43).

Some studies included participant satisfaction as a process indicator (33,56,68,104). While level of satisfaction is not a measure of the effectiveness of an intervention or programme, it can be a useful marker of acceptability and relevance and, therefore, it is often used in training and campaign evaluations. There were three studies that specifically measured the acceptability/feasibility of the intervention/ programme (50,87,111).

Only a small number of evaluation studies included a measure of effectiveness, including implementation effectiveness, programme appropriateness and/or ways in which the intervention or programme contributed to health literacy outcomes. These included indicators on facilitators and barriers, key strengths and limitations, benefits and participant perceptions. Two studies reported on facilitators and barriers to health professionals implementing practice changes within their organizations (following a health literacy training course) (33,104), and one focused more broadly on the facilitators and barriers of implementing a programme as part of the evaluation (35). One study reported on programme strengths and limitations (35), while three studies reported on participant perceptions (which is also likely to provide some information on strengths and limitations) (40,46,56). Two studies reported on benefits of the intervention (33,56). Only one study on a health education intervention targeted at a culturally and linguistically diverse population specifically evaluated the cultural appropriateness of the intervention (52).

2.5 Partnerships and coordination for health literacy measurement

Many of the studies in this report assessed health literacy interventions using experimental research designs; therefore, details on the partnerships and coordination mechanisms were often not described. As such, the roles and responsibilities for data collection and analysis and the accountability mechanisms in place for reporting progress were not clear.

Based on the detail that was provided in some studies, measurement of health literacy interventions often involved multisectoral partnerships, the most common of which were academia–school, academia–community and academia–health service partnerships. Partnerships between academic institutions and government departments or bodies were also reported, while a small number of studies involved corporate or private sector partnerships. The roles and responsibilities of the personnel involved in these studies were generally not described, though some studies did describe joint responsibility for data collection, for example academia–school or academia–health service partnerships in which teachers and clinicians, respectively, led the data collection while the academic researchers undertook data analysis.

One example of a high-level, multisectoral partnership and coordination for evaluation was the national Skilled for Health Programme in the United Kingdom (35), which utilized a multilevel evaluation where a national evaluation team undertook the national evaluation of the programme as well providing technical support for the local evaluations carried out by personnel at the project site.

Another example was the MiMi programme in Germany (36), which was implemented and evaluated through multisectoral partnerships involving academic institutions and local health and community organizations (Case study 3).

Case study 3. Partnership and coordination in the MiMi programme

The MiMi programme in Germany aims to make the health system more accessible to migrants, to increase their health literacy and empower them through a participatory process (36). To achieve this, intercultural mediators are recruited and trained to provide education to their respective migrant communities on the German health system and related health topics.

The MiMi programme was originally developed at the Ethno-Medical Centre with financial support from BKK Bundesverband (Federal Association of Company Health Insurance Funds) and implemented across four cities in two federal states. The programme has expanded to 46 cities involving more than 100 organizations across municipal health and social service sectors.

The Ethno-Medical Centre in cooperation with the BKK Bundesverband provides overall coordination for MiMi. A key condition of becoming a partner on the programme is that organizations must commit to participating in monitoring and evaluation activities to standardize and maintain the quality of the programme.

Evaluation of MiMi occurs at two levels. First, local evaluation of training activities is conducted by partner organizations using standardized questionnaires (pre–post) for trainees and trainers. Secondly, systematic evaluation funded by the German Government is undertaken by the Ethno-Medical Centre in partnership with a medical school, public health service and department of social psychiatry to assess qualitatively (i.e. with interviews and working groups) the use and benefits of the programme for a broad range of stakeholders, as well as to assess the cost–effectiveness of the programme in various settings.

Annual evaluation reports on the programme are developed and published on the MiMi programme website.

In two small-scale health literacy projects, the Roma Men's Training Diversion and Health Literacy Programme (39) and the Action on Health Literacy in Stoke-on-Trent (40), an external evaluation consultant was commissioned to evaluate project processes and outcomes, with support for data collection provided by those partners involved in programme implementation. However, the specific roles and responsibilities of stakeholders under this arrangement were not specified.

2.6 Facilitators and barriers to health literacy measurement

Only a few studies described facilitators and barriers to measuring health literacy or evaluating health literacy interventions or programmes. These can be broadly grouped as skills and capacity of personnel, partnerships, time and budget constraints, and data collection methods and design.

2.6.1 Skills and capacity of personnel

Skills and capacity of personnel was described as both a barrier and a facilitator in some studies. For example, in the evaluation of the United Kingdom Skilled for Health Programme, a lead national evaluation team was established to provide support for local evaluations at project sites. By providing evaluation training activities and one-to-one support to project sites with all aspects of evaluation design and implementation, the skills and capacity of local workers were strengthened for their project evaluations as part of the larger national evaluation. However, the authors noted that it was challenging to provide an equal level of support to all project sites because of the rolling nature of implementation of the programme, which meant that some sites were provided with more intensive support and, therefore, did have greater evaluation capacity than others (35).

Similarly, in an evaluation of a Swedish sexual health programme for migrants, the interpreters were involved in delivering focus groups to ensure that people from diverse language groups could participate and share their experiences. However, the authors acknowledged that, despite working with professional interpreters with experience in the health sector, the interpreters had varying levels of experience, which may have resulted in the meaning of some discussions being lost during the translation process (34).

Another study conducted in Australia indicated that having a skilled evaluation team was a key strength of a qualitative evaluation undertaken to assess a health literacy training course, as it increased the rigour and reliability of the findings (33).

2.6.2 Partnerships

Partnership was identified as a key facilitator of monitoring and evaluation, particularly for national programmes or large multisite programmes. For example, the MiMi programme noted that a partnership between the lead (coordination) organization and a medical school, public health service and department of social psychiatry enabled the programme to draw on the experiences and expertise of skilled researchers and evaluators to ensure that evaluation was undertaken effectively (36). Likewise, the establishment of a national evaluation team involving multiple partners was described as a key strength and enabler of the United Kingdom Skilled for Health Programme, as it enabled a coordinated and consistent approach to evaluation across multiple sites (35).

In the evaluation of the depression awareness campaign for gay men, a partnership between a university, a gay community-based organization and an HIV/AIDS service organization in Switzerland enabled the development, modification and implementation of a population health survey containing measurement domains and indicators relevant for a range of stakeholders and purposes (68).

2.6.3 Time and budget constraints

Time constraints were described as a key barrier to undertaking evaluation in a number of studies. For example, the authors reported that "limited time available for data collection" restricted the sample size of participants in the Swedish sexual health education programme, which resulted in less than half of the participants who consented to participate in the evaluation being interviewed (68). Other studies noted that a lack of time for data collection had a negative effect on the richness of data obtained, or the comprehensiveness of the evaluation overall (41,46). In the Skilled for Health evaluation it was noted that insufficient time and resources were allocated to evaluation activities at a local level through a lack of clarity about the roles and responsibilities of project sites in evaluating their projects (35).

2.6.4 Data collection methods and design

The use of qualitative methods (such as interviews and focus groups) was described as both a strength and a limitation when evaluating health literacy interventions or programmes (34,45–47). They were widely acknowledged as a useful and effective method for gaining rich, in-depth insights into people's experiences and perspectives. They were also shown to be useful for understanding cultural and contextual factors (34,46,48). However, it was also acknowledged that qualitative methods do not allow for a formal assessment of health literacy (34,48) and it can be more challenging to interpret the results (46). Results are more open to the interpretation and biases of evaluators, and it can be more difficult to replicate the analysis in future studies (46). In addition, qualitative methods are more resource intensive and, consequently, sample sizes are often small, which can limit the generalizability of the findings to other population groups and settings (34,48).

Similar facilitators and barriers were described for the use of mixed-methods approaches; however, these were generally considered to be useful and effective for evaluation. For example, mixed-methods provided deeper insights and allowed for the contextualization of quantitative assessments (48,49). They also enabled a more comprehensive understanding of experiences and outcomes from multiple perspectives (45). Some studies also noted that participatory approaches are useful for engaging and empowering communities to have a voice through evaluations and a more meaningful role in co-producing knowledge and evidence building (40,42,47).

Another issue identified was the need to collect demographic and geographical data as part of evaluations. Failure to collect demographic data means the results cannot be aggregated according to characteristics known to play a role in health literacy (i.e. age, sex, socioeconomic status, languages spoken), which also has implications for predicting the effectiveness and appropriateness of programmes and interventions for specific groups in future programmes (36,47).

Timing and frequency of data collection were also identified as potential issues or barriers. In pre–post designs where data are collected immediately or shortly after an intervention, it is harder to measure and understand the long-term or sustained health literacy outcomes of interventions and programmes (45,47). One study that used a longitudinal design acknowledged that it enabled an exploration and understanding of the factors that contribute to development of health literacy over time, but also that it was challenging to maintain the engagement of participants in a long-term study and that the attrition rate increased (49).

2.6.5 Other facilitators

Other key facilitators identified were

- the use of conceptual health literacy frameworks to guide programme evaluation (42);
- the development of evaluation guides including step-by-step instructions and standardized evaluation tools (25);

- clarity around roles and responsibilities in evaluation activities and appropriate allocation of resources (35);
- continuous monitoring to enable the early identification of areas for improvement (49); and
- government funding to support the evaluation of national programmes (35,36).

2.7 Resources and scalability

The level of resources (financial and human) required to undertake an evaluation was not specified in the studies identified for this report; however, evidence from the two studies that reported on national programmes suggests that the level of investment should match the scale and complexity of the programme being implemented and needs to be considered as part of initial programme planning and design (35,36). Some small-scale programmes commissioned an external evaluator to undertake the evaluation; however, the cost involved/funding available to complete the evaluation was not specified.

The scalability of health literacy measures and tools was also not specified in the studies in this report. Many of the studies related to small-scale health literacy interventions or programmes in clinical or community-based settings; consequently the feasibility of scaling the measurement approaches for use at the international, national and subnational levels is not clear.

2.8 Evaluation of health literacy in the WHO European Region

There were 19 studies conducted in the WHO European Region (34–36,38–40,48–50,57–59,67–72,105), almost half of which reported on evaluation activities (34–36,38–40,48–50). The only three national programme evaluations identified for this report were undertaken in Europe: two of these used a mixed-methods approach (35,36) and one used only a qualitative method (34). While there were no national evaluation frameworks identified, there was evidence of the use of both the Sørensen et al. (49) and the Nutbeam (34) health literacy models to inform evaluation design and data collection tools.

Some studies, including three conducted in the Russian Federation, developed custom surveys or instruments to undertake an intervention assessment (58,59,69,71).

There were five studies that used a general health literacy instrument to evaluate a programme or intervention, including AAHLS, HLS-EU, STOFHLA, the Critical Nutrition Literacy Scale, and the Health Literacy in School-aged Children Instrument, the latter of which was the only general health literacy tool developed specifically for use with young people/children identified in this report. The findings showed that self-report health literacy instruments were used more frequently than test-based measures, and in most instances the instruments were used as part of a mixed-methods approach.

The domains and indicators measured in the WHO European Region for personal and mental health literacy were consistent with those measured globally but there were no studies identified that evaluated digital or organizational health literacy as part of a programme or intervention.

The studies conducted in the WHO European Region provided the strongest evidence on the involvement of multisectoral partnerships for coordinating evaluation, particularly two studies on national programmes (the Skilled for Health Programme in the United Kingdom and the MiMi programme in Germany (35,36)).

Finally, the evaluation of the Austrian ÖPGK provided the only evidence on evaluation of a partnership and how this can assess the functions, governance mechanisms and effectiveness of partnerships/alliances that are established to oversee the implementation and monitoring of health literacy policies (38).

3. DISCUSSION

3.1 Strengths and limitations of this review

To the best of our knowledge, this is the first evidence synthesis on approaches for measuring the implementation of health literacy policies, programmes and interventions at the national, regional and organizational levels. A rigorous search strategy was used to identify relevant studies in peer-reviewed literature in English, French, German, Russian and Spanish, with search terms informed by native speakers of the search languages. In addition, experts in health literacy across international networks were contacted for other material. The search strategy was global to enable identification of as many health literacy measures as possible.

A key limitation of the review was that the grey literature search was conducted in English only, which is likely to have excluded some important evaluation studies relevant to the WHO European Region. In addition, as the review focused on studies that evaluated health literacy policies, programmes and interventions, population survey studies undertaken to inform the development of policies in the WHO European Region (and important for future monitoring and evaluation) were not included. However, the measures used in these population surveys, such as the HLS-EU (131), have been used to evaluate/measure programmes and interventions and are reported here.

The report did not include a quality assessment of the studies and their approaches to evaluation and monitoring, nor did it make judgements about whether the data collection tools used in these studies actually measured health literacy. Studies containing measures of health literacy were included on the basis that the authors considered the intervention or programme to be about an aspect of health literacy, and deemed the tools they used to be a measure of health literacy.

3.2 Methodological challenges for health literacy measurement

There are a number of methodological challenges relating to the measurement of health literacy. While there is consensus about the broad definition of health literacy, ideas about suitable domains and priority areas are still being developed. There is no single widely accepted indicator set available. However, there is increased interest in health literacy measurement and there are promising developments, such as

WHO's M-POHL Network (9). The Network will facilitate agreement on indicator sets for regional studies and support international comparability. As indicators sets are developed, however, terminology and concept issues, as well as the contextual and cultural character of the concept, must be considered. Translation and cultural adaptation of health literacy measures into different languages and settings must be consistent and of a high standard (132).

Many of the tools currently used to measure health literacy have been designed to measure functional health literacy and, therefore, measure a limited range of domains (in some cases only one). This is particularly the case for tools that involve test-based measures of health literacy, which, consequently, may not be suitable or feasible for use in monitoring at population/national level. Self-report measures are generally easier to administer, measure a wider range of health literacy domains and have proved to be suitable and feasible for population/national monitoring (131). However, they may lack empirical grounding (133). There are two key issues with self-report measures. First, most of the evidence (predictive validity) for the relevance of health literacy in relation to health outcomes of individuals is derived from test-based measures. Secondly, self-report tools cannot differentiate between the actual skills of individuals and the sociological factors that influence their perceptions of their skills, such as the social desirability effect (134). Studies that have directly compared perceived perception-based with test-based skills have shown poor predictive validity (135).

In addition, many of the validated health literacy instruments are not publicly available, which can limit their use in monitoring and evaluation activities. Many currently also lack sensitivity for cultural or contextual factors. However, the development of international indicator sets, combined with high-quality translation and cultural adaptation where required, will do much to mitigate this. Consideration should also be given to using such tools in combination with qualitative methods to provide a more in-depth, contextualized understanding of people's health literacy capacities.

Finally, methodological challenges are introduced when different conceptual paradigms are considered. For example, individual, public and organizational health literacy concepts and measures have developed as part of a coherent framework of thinking in the health literacy field and include aspects of skills. By comparison, areas such as mental health literacy have developed concepts separately, with a focus on knowledge and attitudes, and often without measurement of skills. Successful evaluation is dependent on clarity about the conceptual paradigm within which the study is sited, the indicators expected to change as a result of any intervention or activity, and the best measurement tools to capture that change.

3.3 National and regional evaluation and monitoring

The review did not identify any policies, programmes or interventions that had been evaluated using national evaluation frameworks or datasets. Evaluation and monitoring frameworks covering a comprehensive range of domains and indicators should be developed to enable consistent population monitoring at the national and subnational levels and produce comparable findings on health literacy across and between countries. The health literacy domains and indicators measured in the WHO European Region were consistent with those measured globally, including for personal health literacy and for mental health literacy. The WHO European Region is in a good position to develop a region-wide approach. The European Health Literacy Project (2) and the resulting HLS-EU (7) started this process, which was followed by a mandate and commitment from WHO European Region Member States to create an international version of HLS-EU. This led to the creation of the M-POHL Network, which is intended to support development of systematic measurement procedures that will be effective across the Member States of the Region and beyond in the future (9).

As health literacy is a relational and context-specific concept, collecting geographical and demographic data (such as age, gender, socioeconomic status, ethnicity and languages spoken) as part of national monitoring and evaluation of programmes will improve the identification of health literacy capacities across population groups to support the development and implementation of policies, programmes and interventions that are tailored to the varying needs of diverse population groups (34–36,39,40).

More evaluation of policies and programmes is needed to improve understanding of the extent to which, and ways in which, health literacy programmes build health literacy skills, particularly for population groups with limited health literacy or those most likely to be impacted by barriers to health literacy, including access to health information and services (34,36,39,40). Efforts to increase the health literacy of both individuals and health-care organizations will contribute to achieving the Sustainable Development Goals (136). In 2019, the WHO Regional Office for Europe and a group of Member States organized a workshop to consider the development, implementation and evaluation of health literacy initiatives across the Region to support the prevention and control of noncommunicable diseases (137). From this, the WHO European Action Network on Health Literacy for Prevention and Control of Noncommunicable Diseases was launched to support individual and collective capacity in the Region for informed decision-making regarding noncommunicable diseases.

The report findings suggest that mixed-methods approaches are likely to be the most effective for evaluating policies, programmes and interventions as they enable a formal assessment of health literacy using quantitative instruments coupled with a more nuanced understanding of the contextual factors that influence health literacy capacities. In addition, the combined use of quantitative and qualitative methods to evaluate the implementation of policies and programmes provides decision-makers with a better understanding of their effectiveness, appropriateness, sustainability and feasibility for further roll-out or expansion.

Increasing the use of participatory methods in evaluation activities is also likely to increase engagement with vulnerable and marginalized population groups and empower them to have a role in the development of evidence and measures that are culturally and contextually relevant. This was highlighted in some studies in this report (40,42,47), and participatory methods are increasingly being used and encouraged in studies examining health literacy (113,138–140).

3.4 Measurement of organizational health literacy responsiveness

The review found limited evidence of the use of organizational health literacy/responsiveness measures and tools as part of an evaluation of a programme or intervention (27). However, progress can be expected through the future work of the M-POHL Network to develop standards for benchmarking and measuring health literacy responsiveness across health-care organizations and systems in the WHO European Region (9). The Organizational Health Literacy Responsiveness (Org-HLR) self-assessment tool has been developed and piloted in Australia and Denmark and shown to have utility in those countries (29,141). A tool has also been developed by a Viennese team for measuring organizational health literacy in Austrian hospitals (30), and has been taken up by a working group of the WHO-initiated International Network of Health Promoting Hospitals and Health Services for use internationally (27). These approaches and tools may provide a useful basis on which to build organizational health literacy measures more broadly.

3.5 Policy considerations

Based on the findings of this scoping review, the following policy considerations are proposed to strengthen the evaluation and monitoring of health literacy policies and programmes across Member States of the WHO European Region:

- develop indicator sets covering a broad range of health literacy domains that would be effective at both the subnational and national levels, facilitate measurement of population health literacy levels and provide data that could be compared across the Region;
- create measurement tools that are suitable for use across multiple settings and at multiple levels in order to support consistent data gathering on population health literacy in the Region;
- expand the use of qualitative and mixed-methods approaches for evaluating policies, programmes and interventions to enable an in-depth understanding of health literacy capacity and the cultural and contextual factors that influence it;
- increase the engagement of citizens, particularly vulnerable and marginalized communities and other relevant stakeholders, in participatory methods to develop measures of health literacy that are culturally and contextually relevant;
- expand the evaluation of health literacy at the organizational and system levels, including on governance, coordination and partnerships and the contextual factors contributing to health literacy; and
- establish partnerships for monitoring and evaluating health literacy policies and programmes, including with research institutions and organizations involved in the advancement of health literacy research, policy and practice.

4. CONCLUSIONS

Health literacy has been recognized as a means to promote health, reduce the risk of illness and premature death, and promote cost-effective, person-centred, equitable health care. Evaluation and monitoring of health literacy policies and related activities are essential to ensure that they are effective. This report presents what is known about the current approaches to evaluating health literacy policies, programmes and interventions and recommends policy considerations that, if adopted, will support consistent and comparable evaluation and monitoring across the WHO European Region. With initiatives such as the M-POHL Network and the recent WHO European Action Network on Health Literacy for Prevention and Control of Noncommunicable Diseases, the WHO European Region is ideally placed to consider and act upon these policy recommendations to enable citizens and society to achieve better and more equitable health towards the attainment of Sustainable Development Goal 3 (to ensure healthy lives and promote well-being for all at all ages).

REFERENCES

1. Kickbusch I, Pelikan JM, Apfel F, Tsouros AD. Health literacy: the solid facts. Copenhagen: WHO Regional Office for Europe, 2013 (http://www.euro.who.int/__data/assets/pdf_file/0008/190655/e96854.pdf, accessed 9 August 2019).

2. Comparative report on health literacy in eight EU Member States. The European Health Literacy Project 2009–2012. Maastricht: HLS-EU Consortium; 2012 (https://cdn1.sph.harvard.edu/wp-content/uploads/sites/135/2015/09/neu_rev_hls-eu_report_2015_05_13_lit.pdf, accessed 8 August 2019).

3. DAC list of ODA recipients: effective for reporting on 2014, 2015 and 2016 flows. Paris: Development Assistance Committee, Organisation for Economic Co-operation and Development; 2017 (http://www.oecd.org/dac/stats/documentupload/DAC_List_ODA_Recipients2014to2017_flows_En.pdf, accessed 9 August 2019).

4. Pelikan JM, Ganahl K. Measuring health literacy in general populations: primary findings from the HLS-EU Consortium's health literacy assessment effort. In: Logan RA, Sigel ER, editors. Health literacy. Amsterdam: IOS Press; 2017:34–59.

5. Shanghai Declaration on promoting health in the 2030 Agenda for Sustainable Development. In: 9th Global conference on health promotion, 21–24 November, 2016. Shanghai: World Health Organization; 2016 (https://www.who.int/healthpromotion/conferences/9gchp/shanghai-declaration.pdf?ua=1, accessed 12 August 2019).

6. Sørensen K, Karuranga S, Denysiuk E, McLernon L. Health literacy and social change: exploring networks and interests groups shaping the rising global health literacy movement. Glob Health Promot. 2018;25(4):89–92. doi: https://doi.org/10.1177/1757975918798366.

7. Pelikan JM, Ganahl K, Van den Broucke S, Sørensen K. Measuring health literacy in Europe: introducing the European Health Literacy Survey Questionnaire (HLS-EU-Q). In: Okan O, Bauer U, Levin-Zamir D, Pinheiro P, Sørensen K, editors. International handbook of health literacy research: policy and practice across the lifespan. Bristol: Policy Press; 2019:115–38.

8. European Health Information Initiative (EHII). Copenhagen: WHO Regional Office for Europe; 2019 (http://www.euro.who.int/en/data-and-evidence/european-health-information-initiative-ehii, accessed 9 August 2019).

9. Dietscher C, Pelikan J, Bobek J, Nowak P. The Action Network on Measuring Population and Organizational Health Literacy (M-POHL): a network under the umbrella of the WHO European Health Information Initiative (EHII). Public Health Panorama. 2019;5(1):65–71 (http://www.euro.who.int/__data/assets/pdf_file/0010/398341/short-comm-health-literacy-eng.pdf?ua=1, accessed 9 August 2019).

10. Rowlands G, Russell S, O'Donnell A, Kaner E, Trezona A, Rademakers J et al. What is the evidence on existing policies and linked activities and their effectiveness for improving health literacy at national, regional and organizational levels in the WHO European Region? Copenhagen: WHO Regional Office for Europe; 2018 (Health Evidence Network (HEN) synthesis report 57; http://www.euro.who.int/__data/assets/pdf_file/0006/373614/Health-evidence-network-synthesis-WHO-HEN-Report-57.pdf?ua=1, accessed 10 August 2019).

11. Sørensen K, Van den Broucke S, Fullam J, Doyle G, Pelikan J, Slonska Z et al. Health literacy and public health: a systematic review and integration of definitions and models. BMC Public Health. 2012;12:80. doi: 10.1186/1471-2458-12-80.

12. Mancuso JM. Assessment and measurement of health literacy: an integrative review of the literature. Nurs Health Sci. 2009;11(1):77–89. doi: 10.1111/j.1442-2018.2008.00408.x.

13. Paasche-Orlow MK, Wolf MS. The causal pathways linking health literacy with health outcomes. Am J Health Behav. 2007;31(suppl 1):S19–26. doi: 10.5555/ajhb.2007.31.supp.S19.

14. Nutbeam D. Health literacy as a public health goal: a challenge for contemporary health education and communication strategies into the 21st century. Health Promot Int. 2000;15(3):259–67. doi: 10.1080/10810730.2017.1417515.

15. Freedman DA, Bess KD, Tucker HA, Boyd DL, Tuchman AM, Wallston KA. Public health literacy defined. Am J Prev Med. 2009;36(5):446–51. doi: 10.1016/j.amepre.2009.02.001.

16. Nutbeam D. The evolving concept of health literacy. Soc Sci Med. 2008;67(12):2072–8. doi: 10.1016/j.socscimed.2008.09.050.

17. Norman CD, Skinner HA. eHealth literacy: essential skills for consumer health in a networked world. J Med Internet Res. 2006;8(2):e9. doi: 10.2196/jmir.8.2.e9.

18. Jorm AF, Korten AE, Jacomb PA, Christensen H, Rodgers B, Pollitt P. "Mental health literacy": a survey of the public's ability to recognise mental disorders and their beliefs about the effectiveness of treatment. Med J Aust. 1997;166(4):182–6. doi: 10.5555/ajhb.2007.31.supp.S19.

19. Kutcher S, Wei Y, Morgan C. Successful application of a Canadian mental health curriculum resource by usual classroom teachers in significantly and sustainably improving student mental health literacy. Can J Psychiatry Rev. 2015;60(12):580–6. doi: 10.1177/070674371506001209.

20. Parker RM, Hernandez LM. What makes an organization health literate? J Health Commun. 2012;17(5):624–7. doi: 10.1080/10810730.2012.685806.

21. Rudd R, Anderson JE. The health literacy environment of hospitals and health centers: making your healthcare facility literacy friendly. Boston (MA): Harvard School of Public Health; 2006.

22. Meggetto E, Ward B, Issacs A. What's in a name? An overview of organizational health literacy terminology. Aust Health Rev. 2017;42(1):21–30. doi: 10.1071/AH17077.

23. Palumbo R. Designing health-literate health care organizations: a literature review. Health Care Manage Rev. 2016;29(3):79–87. doi: 10.1177/0951484816639741.

24. Brach C. The journey to become a health literate organization: a snapshot of health system improvement. Stud Health Technol Inform. 2017;240:203–37. PMID: 28972519.

25. Farmanova E, Bonneville L, Bouchard L. Organizational health literacy: review of theories, frameworks, guides and implementation issues. Inquiry. 2018;55:1–17. doi: 10.1177/0046958018757848.

26. Lloyd JE, Song HJ, Dennis SM, Dunbar N, Harris E, Harris MF. A paucity of strategies for developing health literate organizations: a systematic review. PLOS One. 2018;13(4):e0195018. doi: 10.1371/journal.pone.0195018.

27. Pelikan JM. Health-literate healthcare organizations. In: Okan O, Bauer U, Levin-Zamir D, Sørensen K, editors. International handbook of health literacy research: practice and policy across the lifespan. Bristol: Policy Press; 2019:539–54.

28. Trezona A, Dodson S, Osborne RH. Development of the Organisational Health Literacy Responsiveness (Org-HLR) Framework in collaboration with health and social services professionals. BMC Health Serv Res. 2017;17(1):513. doi: 10.1186/s12913-017-2465-z.

29. Trezona A, Dodson S, Osborne RH. Development of the Organisational Health Literacy Responsiveness (Org-HLR) self-assessment tool and process. BMC Health Serv Res. 2018;18(1):694. doi: 10.1186/s12913-018-3499-6.

30. Dietscher C, Pelikan JM. Health literate hospitals and healthcare organizations: results from an Austrian feasibility study on the self-assessment of organizational health literacy in hospitals. In: Schaeffer D, Pelikan JM, editors. Health literacy: Forschungsstand und Perspektiven. Gottingen: Hogrefe; 2017:303–14.

31. Brach C, Keller D, Hernandez LM, Baur C, Parker R, Dreyer B et al. Ten attributes of health literate health care organizations; a discussion paper. Washington (DC): Institute of Medicine; 2012.

32. Health literacy tool shed. Boston (MA): Boston University; 2019 (https://healthliteracy.bu.edu, accessed 10 August 2019).

33. Naccarella L, Greenstock L. Evaluation of the Centre for Culture, Ethnicity and Health 2013 health literacy course. Melbourne: Australian Health Workforce Institute, University of Melbourne; 2013.

34. Svensson P, Carlzen K, Agardh A. Exposure to culturally sensitive sexual health information and impact on health literacy: a qualitative study among newly arrived refugee women in Sweden. Cult Health Sex. 2017;19(7):752–66. doi: 10.1080/13691058.2016.

35. Evaluation of the second phase of the Skilled for Health Programme. London: The Tavistock Institute and Shared Intelligence; 2009.

36. Salman R, Weyers S. MiMi project: with migrants for migrants. In: Koller T, editor. Poverty and social exclusion in the WHO European Region: health systems respond. Copenhagen: WHO Regional Office for Europe; 2010:52–63 (http://www.euro.who.int/__data/assets/pdf_file/0006/115485/E94018.pdf, accessed 13 August 2019).

37. Bond KS, Jorm AF, Kitchener BA, Reavley NJ. Mental health first aid training for Australian medical and nursing students: an evaluation study. BMC Psychol. 2015;3(1):11. doi: 10.1186/s40359-015-0069-0.

38. Gutknecht-Gmeiner M, Capellaro M. Evaluation der Österreichischen Plattform Gesundheitskompetenz (ÖPGK). Vienna: Humburg; 2016.

39. Scullion G. Evaluation of the Atelier Roma Men's Training, Diversion and Health Literacy Programme. Dublin: Health Service Executive; 2016.

40. Estacio EV. Action on health literacy in Stoke-on-Trent: engaging south Asian men and young men with diabetes. Newcastle-under-Lyme: Keele University; 2012.

41. Grace S, Horstmanshof L. A realist evaluation of a regional dementia health literacy project. Health Expect. 2019;22(3):426–34. doi: 10.1111/hex.12862.

42. Simonds VW, Kim FL, LaVeaux D, Pickett V, Milakovich J, Cummins J. Guardians of the living water: using a health literacy framework to evaluate a child as change agent intervention. Health Educ Behav. 2019;46(2):349–59. doi: 10.1177/1090198118798676.

43. Parker SM, Stocks N, Nutbeam D, Thomas L, Denney-Wilson E, Zwar N et al. Preventing chronic disease in patients with low health literacy using eHealth and teamwork in primary healthcare: protocol for a cluster randomised controlled trial. BMJ Open. 2018;8(6):e023239. doi: 10.1136/bmjopen-2018-023239.

44. Nash R, Elmer S, Thomas K, Osborne R, MacIntyre K, Shelley B et al. HealthLit4Kids study protocol; crossing boundaries for positive health literacy outcomes. BMC Public Health. 2018;18(1):690. doi: 10.1186/s12889-018-5558-7.

45. Davis LF, Ramirez-Andreotta MD, McLain JET, Kilungo A, Abrell L, Buxner S. Increasing environmental health literacy through contextual learning in communities at risk. Int J Environ Res Pub Health. 2018;15(10):pii. doi: 10.3390/ijerph15102203.

46. Vollmer Dahlke D, Fair K, Hong YA, Kellstedt D, Ory MG. Adolescent and young adult cancer survivorship educational programming: a qualitative evaluation. JMIR Cancer. 2017;3(1):e3. doi: 10.2196/cancer.5821.

47. Elmer S, Bridgman H, Williams A, Bird M, Murray S, Jones R et al. Evaluation of a health literacy program for chronic conditions. Health Lit Res Pract. 2017;1(3):e100–8. doi: 10.3928/24748307-20170523-01.

48. Sykes S, Wills J. Challenges and opportunities in building critical health literacy. Glob Health Promot. 2018;1757975918789352. doi: 10.1177/1757975918789352 (Epub ahead of print).

49. McKenna VB, Sixsmith J, Barry MM. A qualitative study of the development of health literacy capacities of participants attending a community-based cardiovascular health programme. Int J Environ Res Public Health. 2018;15(6):pii. doi: 10.3390/ijerph15061157.

50. Chisholm K, Patterson P, Torgerson C, Turner E, Jenkinson D, Birchwood M. Impact of contact on adolescents' mental health literacy and stigma: the SchoolSpace cluster randomised controlled trial. BMJ Open. 2016;6(2):e009435. doi: 10.1136/bmjopen-2015-009435.

51. Vella SA, Swann C, Batterham M, Boydell KM, Eckermann S, Fogarty A et al. Ahead of the game protocol: a multi-component, community sport-based program targeting prevention, promotion and early intervention for mental health among adolescent males. BMC Public Health. 2018;18(1):390. doi: 10.1186/s12889-018-5319-7.

52. Calderón JL, Shaheen M, Hays RD, Fleming ES, Norris KC, Baker RS. Improving diabetes health literacy by animation. Diabetes Educ. 2014;40(3):361–72. doi: 10.1177/0145721714527518.

53. Ansell M, Tennant MR, Piazza V, Cottler LB. Piloting consumer health information services in collaboration with a community research engagement program. Med Ref Serv Q. 2017;36(4):348–61. doi: 10.1080/02763869.2017.1369283.

54. Faruqi N, Stocks N, Spooner C, El Haddad N, Harris MF. Research protocol: management of obesity in patients with low health literacy in primary health care. BMC Obes. 2015;2:5. doi: 10.1186/s40608-015-0036-6.

55. McCaffery KJ, Morony S, Muscat DM, Smith SK, Shepherd HL, Dhillon HM et al. Evaluation of an Australian health literacy training program for socially disadvantaged adults attending basic education classes: study protocol for a cluster randomised controlled trial. BMC Public Health. 2016;16:454. doi: 10.1186/s12889-016-3034-9.

56. Muscat DM, Smith S, Dhillon HM, Morony S, Davis EL, Luxford K et al. Incorporating health literacy in education for socially disadvantaged adults: an Australian feasibility study. Int J Equity Health. 2016;15:84. doi: 10.1186/s12939-016-0373-1.

57. Svensson B, Hansson L. Effectiveness of mental health first aid training in Sweden. A randomized controlled trial with a six-month and two-year follow-up. PLOS One. 2014;9(6):e100911. doi: 10.1371/journal.pone.0100911.

58. Kalinina AM, Gomova TA, Kushunina DV, Soin IA, Izmaylova OV, Khudyakov MB. Профилактическая активность пациентов поликлиник как важный фактор эффективности диспансеризации и диспансерного наблюдения: региональный опыт [Prophylactic activity of outpatients as an important factor of the efficiency of prophylactic medical examination and case follow-up]. Prev Med. 2015;18:4–10. doi: 10.17116/profmed20151824-10 (in Russian).

59. Maksimova ZV, Fasakhova DA, Glukhovskaya SV. Профилактика в клинической практике: взгляд врачей первичного звена [Prevention in clinical practice: the views of primary health care physicians]. Prev Med. 2014;17:49–54 (in Russian).

60. Chi H-Y, Chang F-C, Huang L-J, Lee C-H, Pan Y-C, Yeh M-K. Enhancing teachers' medication literacy and teaching through school-pharmacist partnership in Taiwan. Drugs: Educ Prev Polic. 2018;25(6):491–9. doi: 10.1080/09687637.2017.1321620.

61. Kreslake JM, Price KM, Sarfaty M. Developing effective communication materials on the health effects of climate change for vulnerable groups: a mixed methods study. BMC Public Health. 2016;16:946. doi: 10.1186/s12889-016-3546-3.

62. Swartz K, Musci RJ, Beaudry MB, Heley K, Miller L, Alfes C et al. School-based curriculum to improve depression literacy among US secondary school students: a randomized effectiveness trial. Am J Public Health. 2017;107(12):1970–6. doi: 10.2105/AJPH.2017.304088.

63. Brown V, Russell M, Ginter A, Braun B, Little L, Pippidis M et al. Smart choice health insurance(©): a new, interdisciplinary program to enhance health insurance literacy. Health Promot Pract. 2016;17(2):209–16. doi: 10.1177/1524839915620393.

64. Thorsteinsson EB, Bhullar N, Williams E, Loi NM. Schizophrenia literacy: the effects of an educational intervention on populations with and without prior health education. J Ment Health. 2019;28(3):229–37. doi: 10.1080/09638237.2018.1521923.

65. Nsangi A, Semakula D, Oxman AD, Oxman M, Rosenbaum S, Austvoll-Dahlgren A et al. Does the use of the Informed Healthcare Choices (IHC) primary school resources improve the ability of grade 5 children in Uganda to assess the trustworthiness of claims about the effects of treatments: protocol for a cluster-randomised trial. Trials. 2017;18(1):223. doi: 10.1186/s13063-017-1958-8.

66. Semakula D, Nsangi A, Oxman M, Austvoll-Dahlgren A, Rosenbaum S, Kaseje M et al. Can an educational podcast improve the ability of parents of primary school children to assess the reliability of claims made about the benefits and harms of treatments: study protocol for a randomised controlled trial. Trials. 2017;18(1):31. doi: 10.1186/s13063-016-1745-y.

67. Bjørnsen H, Ringdal R, Espnes G, Eilertsen M, Moksnes U. Exploring MEST: a new universal teaching strategy for school health services to promote positive mental health literacy and mental wellbeing among Norwegian adolescents. BMC Health Serv Res. 2018;18(1):1001. doi: 10.1186/s12913-018-3829-8.

68. Wang J, Häusermann M, Berrut S, Weiss MG. The impact of a depression awareness campaign on mental health literacy and mental morbidity among gay men. J Affect Disord. 2013;150(2):306–12. doi: 10.1016/j.jad.2013.04.011.

69. Casañas R, Arfuch V-M, Castellví P, Gil J-J, Torres M, Pujol A et al. "EspaiJove.net": a school-based intervention programme to promote mental health and eradicate stigma in the adolescent population – study protocol for a cluster randomised controlled trial. BMC Public Health. 2018;18(1):939. doi: 10.1186/s12889-018-5855-1.

70. Hansson L, Markström U. The effectiveness of an anti-stigma intervention in a basic police officer training programme: a controlled study. BMC Psychiatry. 2014;14:55. doi: 10.1186/1471-244X-14-55.

71. Shamalov NA, Shetova IM, Anisimova AV, Gordeev MN, Anisimov KV. Повышение информированности населения о симптомах инсульта [Increasing public awareness of stroke symptoms. The program of the Moscow Department of Health]. Prev Med. 2018;21:S21–30 (in Russian).

72. Kudryavtseva NG, Nikolenko NV, Sakharova OI, Vasilchenko VL, Tumanova SA, Gorbunova EV et al. Отдаленная эффективность обучающей программы для пациентов с протезами клапанов сердца в повышении приверженности к лечению и качества жизни [Long-term efficiency of training programme for patients with artificial heart valves to improve the adherence to treatment and quality of life]. Cardiol Cardiovasc Surg. 2017;10(4):13–18. doi: 10.17116/kardio201710413-18 (in Russian).

73. Perry Y, Petrie K, Buckley H, Cavanagh L, Clarke D, Winslade M et al. Effects of a classroom-based educational resource on adolescent mental health literacy: a cluster randomized controlled trial. J Adolesc. 2014;37(7):1143–51. doi: 10.1016/j.adolescence.2014.08.001.

74. Nahm E-S, Zhu S, Bellantoni M, Keldsen L, Russomanno V, Rietschel M et al. The effects of a theory-based patient portal e-learning program for older adults with chronic illnesses. Telemed J E Health. 2018. doi: 10.1089/tmj.2018.0184 (Epub ahead of print).

75. Shensa A, Phelps-Tschang J, Miller E, Primack BA. A randomized crossover study of web-based media literacy to prevent smoking. Health Educ Res. 2016;31(1):48–59. doi: 10.1093/her/cyv062.

76. Fiscella K, Boyd M, Brown J, Carroll J, Cassells A, Corales R et al. Activation of persons living with HIV for treatment, the great study. BMC Public Health. 2015;15:1056. doi: 10.1186/s12889-015-2382-1.

77. Yee LM, Wolf M, Mullen R, Bergeron AR, Cooper Bailey S, Levine R et al. A randomized trial of a prenatal genetic testing interactive computerized information aid. Prenat Diagn. 2014;34(6):552–7. doi: 10.1002/pd.4347.

78. Unger JB, Cabassa LJ, Molina GB, Contreras S, Baron M. Evaluation of a fotonovela to increase depression knowledge and reduce stigma among Hispanic adults. J Immigr Minor Health. 2013;15(2):398–406. doi: 10.1007/s10903-012-9623-5.

79. Tavakoly Sany SB, Peyman N, Behzhad F, Esmaeily H, Taghipoor A, Ferns G. Health providers' communication skills training affects hypertension outcomes. Med Teach. 2018;40(2):154–63. doi: 10.1080/0142159X.2017.1395002.

80. Kim KB, Han HR, Huh B, Nguyen T, Lee H, Kim MT. The effect of a community-based self-help multimodal behavioral intervention in Korean American seniors with high blood pressure. Am J Hypertens. 2014;27(9):1199–208. doi: 10.1093/ajh/hpu041.

81. Uemura K, Yamada M, Okamoto H. Effects of active learning on health literacy and behavior in older adults: a randomized controlled trial. Am J Hypertens. 2018;66(9):1721–9. doi: 10.1111/jgs.15458.

82. Skau JK, Nordin AB, Cheah JC, Ali R, Zainal R, Aris T et al. A complex behavioural change intervention to reduce the risk of diabetes and prediabetes in the pre-conception period in Malaysia: study protocol for a randomised controlled trial. Trials. 2016;17(1):215. doi: 10.1186/s13063-016-1345-x.

83. Jarernsiripornkul N, Chaipichit N, Chumworathayi P, Krska J. Management for improving patients' knowledge and understanding about drug allergy. Pharm Pract (Granada). 2015;13(1):513. PMID: 25883688.

84. Paudel P, Yen PT, Kovai V, Naduvilath T, Ho SM, Giap NV et al. Effect of school eye health promotion on children's eye health literacy in Vietnam. Health Promot Int. 2019;34(1):113–22. doi: 10.1093/heapro/dax065.

85. Lai ESY, Kwok C-L, Wong PWC, Fu K-W, Law Y-W, Yip PSF. The effectiveness and sustainability of a universal school-based programme for preventing depression in Chinese adolescents: a follow-up study using quasi-experimental design. PLOS One. 2016;11(2):e0149854. doi: 10.1371/journal.pone.0149854.

86. Carroll LN, Smith SA, Thomson NR. Parents as teachers health literacy demonstration project: integrating an empowerment model of health literacy promotion into home-based parent education. Health Promot Int. 2015;16(2):282–90. doi: 10.1177/1524839914538968.

87. Li W, Han LQ, Guo YJ, Sun J. Using WeChat official accounts to improve malaria health literacy among Chinese expatriates in Niger: an intervention study. Malar J. 2016;15(1):567. doi: 10.1186/s12936-016-1621-y.

88. McLuckie A, Kutcher S, Wei Y, Weaver C. Sustained improvements in students' mental health literacy with use of a mental health curriculum in Canadian schools. BMC Psychiatry. 2014;14:379. doi: 10.1186/s12888-014-0379-4.

89. Milin R, Kutcher S, Lewis SP, Walker S, Wei Y, Ferrill N et al. Impact of a mental health curriculum on knowledge and stigma among high school students: a randomized controlled trial. J Am Acad Child Adolesc Psychiatry. 2016;55(5):383–91.e1. doi: 10.1016/j.jaac.2016.02.018.

90. Ravindran AV, Herrera A, da Silva TL, Henderson J, Castrillo ME, Kutcher S. Evaluating the benefits of a youth mental health curriculum for students in Nicaragua: a parallel-group, controlled pilot investigation. Glob Ment Health (Camb). 2018;5:e4. doi: 10.1017/gmh.2017.27.

91. Chu JTW, Whittaker R, Jiang Y, Wadham A, Stasiak K, Shepherd M et al. Evaluation of MyTeen: a SMS-based mobile intervention for parents of adolescents – a randomised controlled trial protocol. BMC Public Health. 2018;5:e4. doi: 10.1186/s12889-018-6132-z.

92. Wong DFK, Lau Y, Kwok S, Wong P, Tori C. Evaluating the effectiveness of mental health first aid program for Chinese People in Hong Kong. Res Soc Work Pract. 2017;27(1):59–67. doi: 10.1177/1049731515585149.

93. Moll SE, Patten S, Stuart H, MacDermid JC, Kirsh B. Beyond silence: a randomized, parallel-group trial exploring the impact of workplace mental health literacy training with healthcare employees. Can J Psychiatry. 2018;63(12):826–33. doi: 10.1177/0706743718766051.

94. Mnatzaganian C, Fricovsky E, Best BM, Singh RF. An interactive, multifaceted approach to enhancing pharmacy students' health literacy knowledge and confidence. Am J Pharm Educ. 2017;81(2):32. doi: 10.5688/ajpe81232.

95. Mohatt NV, Boeckmann R, Winkel N, Mohatt DF, Shore J. Military mental health first aid: development and preliminary efficacy of a community training for improving knowledge, attitudes, and helping behaviors. Mil Med. 2017;182(1):e1576–83. doi: 10.7205/MILMED-D-16-00033.

96. Cartes-Velasquez R, Araya C, Flores R, Luengo L, Castillo F, Bustos A. A motivational interview intervention delivered at home to improve the oral health literacy and reduce the morbidity of Chilean disadvantaged families: a

study protocol for a community trial. BMJ Open. 2017;7(7):e011819. doi: 10.1136/bmjopen-2016-011819.

97. Pagels P, Kindratt T, Arnold D, Brandt J, Woodfin G, Gimpel N. Training family medicine residents in effective communication skills while utilizing promotoras as standardized patients in OSCEs: a health literacy curriculum. Int J Family Med. 2015;2015:129187. doi: 10.1155/2015/129187.

98. Primack BA, Douglas EL, Land SR, Miller E, Fine MJ. Comparison of media literacy and usual education to prevent tobacco use: a cluster-randomized trial. J Sch Health. 2014;84(2):106–15. doi: 10.1111/josh.12130.

99. Zhuang R, Xiang Y, Han T, Yang G-A, Zhang Y. Cell phone-based health education messaging improves health literacy. Afr Health Sci. 2016;16(1):311–18. doi: 10.4314/ahs.v16i1.41.

100. Hjertstedt J, Barnes SL, Sjostedt JM. Investigating the impact of a community-based geriatric dentistry rotation on oral health literacy and oral hygiene of older adults. Gerodontology. 2014;31(4):296–307. doi: 10.1111/ger.12038.

101. Trujillo JM, Figler TA. Teaching and learning health literacy in a doctor of pharmacy program. Am J Pharm Educ. 2015;79(2):27. doi: 10.5688/ajpe79227.

102. Mas FS, Ji M, Fuentes BO, Tinajero J. The health literacy and ESL study: a community-based intervention for Spanish-speaking adults. J Health Commun. 2015;20(4):369–76. doi: 10.1080/10810730.2014.965368.

103. Tai BW, Bae YH, LaRue CE, Law AV. Putting words into action: a simple focused education improves prescription label comprehension and functional health literacy. J Am Pharm Assoc. 2016;56(2):145-2.e3. doi: 10.1016/j.japh.2015.12.010.

104. Green JA, Gonzaga AM, Cohen ED, Spagnoletti CL. Addressing health literacy through clear health communication: a training program for internal medicine residents. Patient Educ Couns. 2014;95(1):76–82. doi: 10.1016/j.pec.2014.01.004.

105. Woods-Townsend K, Bagust L, Barker M, Christodoulou A, Davey H, Godfrey K et al. Engaging teenagers in improving their health behaviours and increasing their interest in science (evaluation of LifeLab Southampton): study protocol for a cluster randomized controlled trial. Trials. 2015;16:372. doi: 10.1186/s13063-015-0890-z.

106. Ayub RA, Jaffery T, Aziz F, Rahmat M. Improving health literacy of women about iron deficiency anemia and civic responsibility of students through service learning. Educ Health (Abingdon). 2015;28(2):130–7. doi: 10.4103/1357-6283.170122.

107. Ishikawa H, Yamaguchi I, Nutbeam D, Kato M, Okuhara T, Okada M et al. Improving health literacy in a Japanese community population: a pilot study to develop an educational programme. Health Expect. 2018;21(4):814–21. doi: 10.1111/hex.12678.

108. St Jean B, Greene Taylor N, Kodama C, Subramaniam M. Assessing the digital health literacy skills of tween participants in a school-library-based after-school program. J Consum Health Internet. 2017;21(1):40–61. doi 10.1080/15398285.2017.1279894.

109. Burns S, Crawford G, Hallett J, Hunt K, Chih HJ, Tilley PJ. What's wrong with John? A randomised controlled trial of mental health first aid (MHFA) training with nursing students. BMC Psychiatry. 2017;17(1):111. doi: 10.1186/s12888-017-1278-2.

110. Lori JR, Ofosu-Darkwah H, Boyd CJ, Banerjee T, Adanu RMK. Improving health literacy through group antenatal care: a prospective cohort study. BMC Pregnancy Childb. 2017;17:1–9. doi: 10.1186/s12884-017-1414-5.

111. Sibeko G, Milligan PD, Roelofse M, Molefe L, Jonker D, Ipser J et al. Piloting a mental health training programme for community health workers in South Africa: an exploration of changes in knowledge, confidence and attitudes. BMC Psychiatry. 2018;18(1):191. doi: 10.1186/s12888-018-1772-1.

112. Milford E, Morrison K, Teutsch C, Nelson BB, Herman A, King M et al. Out of the classroom and into the community: medical students consolidate learning about health literacy through collaboration with Head Start. BMC Med Educ. 2016;16:121. doi: 10.1186/s12909-016-0635-z.

113. Ardiles P, Casteleijn M, Black C, Sørensen K. Using Photovoice as a participatory approach to promote youth health literacy. In: Okan O, Bauer U, Levin-Zamir D, Pinheiro P, Sørensen K, editors. International handbook of health literacy: research, practice and policy across the lifespan. Bristol: Policy Press; 2019:247–60.

114. Parker RM, Baker DW, Williams MV, Nurss JR. The Test of Functional Health Literacy in Adults: a new instrument for measuring patients' literacy skills. J Gen Intern Med. 1995;10(10):537–41. doi: 10.1007/bf02640361.

115. Chinn D, McCarthy C. All Aspects of Health Literacy Scale (AAHLS): developing a tool to measure functional, communicative and critical health literacy in primary healthcare settings. Patient Educ Couns. 2013;90(2):247–53. doi: 10.1016/j.pec.2012.10.019.

116. Baker DW, Williams MV, Parker RM, Gazmararian JA, Nurss J. Development of a brief test to measure functional health literacy. Patient Educ Couns. 1999;38(1):33–42. PMID: 14528569.

117. Osborne RH, Batterham RW, Elsworth GR, Hawkins M, Buchbinder R. The grounded psychometric development and initial validation of the Health Literacy Questionnaire (HLQ). BMC Public Health. 2013;13:658. doi: 10.1186/1471-2458-13-658.

118. Chung S, Nahm ES. Testing reliability and validity of the eHealth Literacy Scale (eHEALS) for older adults recruited online. Comput Inform Nurs. 2015;33(4):150–6. doi: 10.1097/CIN.0000000000000146.

119. Sørensen K, Van den Broucke S, Pelikan JM, Fullam J, Doyle G, Slonska Z et al. Measuring health literacy in populations: illuminating the design and development process of the European Health Literacy Survey Questionnaire (HLS-EU-Q). BMC Public Health. 2013;13:948. doi: 10.1186/1471-2458-13-948.

120. Ishikawa H, Takeuchi T, Yano E. Measuring functional, communicative, and critical health literacy among diabetic patients. Diabetes Care. 2008;31(5):874–9. doi: 10.2337/dc07-1932.

121. Morris N, MacLean CD, Chew LD, Littenberg B. The single item literacy screener: evaluation of a brief instrument to identify limited reading ability. BMC Fam Pract. 2006;7:21–7.

122. Anxiety Literacy Questionnaire [website]. Canberra: Centre for Mental Health Research, Australian National University; 2019 (https://rsph.anu.edu.au/research/tools-resources/anxiety-literacy-questionnaire-lit, accessed 13 August 2019).

123. Depression Literacy Questionnaire [website]. Canberra: Centre for Mental Health Research, Australian National University; 2019 (https://rsph.anu.edu.au/research/tools-resources/depression-literacy-questionnaire-d-lit, accessed 13 August 2019).

124. O'Connor M, Casey L. The Mental Health Literacy Scale (MHLS): a new scale-based measure of mental health literacy. Psychiatry Res. 2015;229(1–2):511–16. doi: 10.1016/j.psychres.2015.05.064.

125. Thornicroft G. Mental health knowledge schedule (MAKS). London: Institute of Psychiatry, King's College London; 2009 (http://www.cles.org.uk/wp-content/uploads/2011/03/Mental-health-knowledge-schedule.pdf, accessed 12 August 2019).

126. Evans-Lacko S, Little K, Meltzer H, Rose D, Rhydderch D, Henderson C et al. Development and psychometric properties of the Mental Health Knowledge Schedule. Can J Psychiatry. 2010;55(7):440–8. doi: 10.1177/070674371005500707.

127. Griffiths KM, Christensen H, Jorm AF, Evans K, Groves C. Effect of web-based depression literacy and cognitive-behavioural therapy interventions on stigmatising attitudes to depression: randomised controlled trial. Br J Psychiatry. 2004;185:342–9. doi: 10.1192/bjp.185.4.342.

128. Gulliver A, Griffiths KM, Christensen H, Mackinnon A, Calear AL, Parsons A et al. Internet-based interventions to promote mental health help-seeking in elite athletes: an exploratory randomized controlled trial. J Med Internet Res. 2012;14(3):e69. doi: 10.2196/jmir.1864.

129. HELLO TAS! toolkit (a toolkit for health literacy learning organisations). Sandy Bay: Tasmanian Council of Social Services; 2019 (https://www.hellotas.org.au, accessed 12 August 2019).

130. Peersman G, Rugg D. Basic terminology and frameworks for monitoring and evaluation. Geneva: Joint United Nations Programme on HIV and AIDS; 2010 (https://www.unaids.org/sites/default/files/sub_landing/files/7_1-Basic-Terminology-and-Frameworks-MEF.pdf, accessed 12 August 2019).

131. Sørensen K, Pelikan JM, Rothlin F, Ganahl K, Slonska Z, Doyle G et al. Health literacy in Europe: comparative results of the European health literacy survey (HLS-EU). Eur J Public Health. 2015;25(6):1053–8. doi: 10.1093/eurpub/ckv043.

132. Andrulis DP, Brach C. Integrating literacy, culture, and language to improve health care quality for diverse populations. Am J Health Behav. 2007;31(suppl 1):S122–33.

133. Pleasant A, Maish C, O'Leary C, Carmona R. Measuring health literacy in adults: an overview and discussion of current tools. In: Okan O, Bauer U, Levin-Zamir D, Pinheiro P, Sørensen K, editors. International handbook of health literacy research: policy and practice across the lifespan. Bristol: Policy Press; 2019:67–82.

134. van de Mortel TF. Faking it: social desirability response bias in self-report research. Aust J Adv Nurs. 2008;25(4):40–8.

135. Mantwill S, Allam A, Camerini AL, Schulz PJ. Validity of three brief health literacy screeners to measure functional health literacy: evidence from five different countries. J Health Commun. 2018;23(2):153–61. doi: 10.1080/10810730.2017.1417515.

136. Transforming our world: the 2030 agenda for sustainable development. New York: United Nations; 2015 (United Nations General Assembly resolution 70/1; http://www.un.org/ga/search/view_doc.asp?symbol=A/RES/70/1&Lang=E, accessed 18 August 2019).

137. Health literacy as a lever to prevent and control NCDs: workshop in Portugal. In: Media centre [website]. Copenhagen: WHO Regional Office for Europe; 2019 (http://www.euro.who.int/en/media-centre/events/events/2019/01/health-literacy-as-a-lever-to-prevent-and-control-ncds-workshop-in-portugal, accessed 12 August 2019).

138. Sykes S, Wills J. Critical health literacy for the marginalised: empirical findings. In: Okan O, Bauer U, Levin-Zamir D, Pinheiro P, Sørensen K, editors. International handbook of health literacy: research, practice and policy across the lifespan. Bristol: Policy Press; 2019:167–82.

139. Bittlingmayer U, Sahrai D. Health literacy for all? Inclusion as a serious challenge for health literacy: the case of disability. In: Okan O, Bauer U, Levin-Zamir D, Pinheiro P, Sørensen K, editors. International handbook of health literacy: research, practice and policy across the lifespan. Bristol: Policy Press; 2019:689–704.

140. Bollweg TM, Okan O. Measuring children's health literacy: current approaches and challenges. In: Okan O, Bauer U, Levin-Zamir D, Pinheiro P, Sørensen K, editors. International handbook of health literacy: research, practice and policy across the lifespan. Bristol: Policy Press; 2019:83–98.

141. Aaby A, Maindal H. Organizational health literacy responsiveness – making organisations fit for diversity. In: 10th European Conference of the International Union for Health Promotion and Education, Trondheim, September 2018 (poster).

ANNEX 1. SEARCH STRATEGY

Databases, websites and other sources

Searches were conducted between 6 January 2019 and 20 January 2019. The following databases were searched for academic peer-reviewed literature in English, French, German and Spanish using defined search terms: CINAHL (Cumulative Index to Nursing and Allied Health Literature), the Cochrane Library, ERIC (Educational Resource Information Centre), MEDLINE, PsychInfo and PubMed. The search for Russian language publications was undertaken in E-library, MediaSphera and Medical Library. An Internet search of grey literature in English was conducted in Google.

The searches were supplemented by findings in HEN report 57 (1) and enquires with experts through the Global Working Group of the International Union for Health Promotion and Education and the M-POHL Network.

Study selection

The results of all database searches were downloaded and combined into a single database. After removing duplicates, the titles and abstracts were screened by two reviewers for eligibility using the inclusion and exclusion criteria described below. Studies were only included if they measured health literacy as part of an evaluation of a policy or programme or in an assessment of an intervention. In order to include as much evidence as possible, published protocols of studies were included if there was no publication relating to a completed study.

Health literacy measurement is undertaken as part of both evaluation studies and measurement studies. In this report, evaluation studies were those that assessed the implementation, acceptability or appropriateness of a programme or intervention (e.g. facilitator and barriers to implementation, strengths and limitations, and recommendations for improvement). Measurement studies were those that assessed the effect of a health literacy intervention using experimental designs such as randomized controlled trials, community-based cluster trials, brief clinical health service interventions or other research-oriented study designs and did not include an assessment of the programme or intervention itself.

Evaluations of programmes and assessments of interventions were included in this report as much of the available evidence on health literacy measurement has been developed through intervention studies (research). These are likely to be useful and relevant in guiding the evaluation and monitoring of national health literacy policies and programmes.

Inclusion and exclusion criteria

Inclusion criteria were:

- published between 1 January 2013 and 31 December 2018;
- published in English, French, German, Russian or Spanish;
- must contain the term health literacy (or equivalent translated terms);
- must contain measures/instruments that are publically available (within the study, via a website or by request to the author);
- health literacy measures had been applied to policy/intervention development and/or evaluation; and
- any geographical area.

Exclusion criteria were:

- editorials, comments, conference abstracts or letters
- studies relating to dyslexia
- studies on general reading and writing
- studies on general education interventions
- studies on readability tools or the assessment of readability of health information
- measures on general literacy/numeracy
- health literacy measures used for research purposes only
- study not sited within a health promotion paradigm.

Search terms

Search terms in English, French, German, Russian and Spanish were used to identify literature. All the relevant terms used in HEN report 57 on health literacy policies and related activities in the WHO European Region (1) were included, but the search was structured with health literacy as the key search term. To limit the number of irrelevant search results, the search was limited to documents including the term health literacy (or equivalent translated terms).

Table A1.1 has the search terms used for the peer-reviewed literature search in English, French, German and Spanish and Table A1.2 the terms used for the search in Russian.

Table A1.1. Search strategy in English, French, German and Spanish

	Terms	Type
	"Health literacy" OR "Littératie en matière de santé" OR Gesundheitskompetenz OR "Alfabetización en salud"	All fields
AND	literacy OR l'alphabétisation OR Lesefähigkeit OR Schreibfähigkeit OR alfabetización OR literate OR alphabète OR lesekundig OR schreibkundig OR alfabetizado OR "reading skills" "compétences en lecture" OR Lesefähigkeiten OR "habilidades de lectura" OR "reading ability" OR "capacité de lecture" OR lesefähigkeit OR "habilidad de lectura" OR "reading level" OR "niveau de lecture" OR lesestufe OR "nivel de lectura" OR "writing level" OR "niveau d'écriture" OR schreibstufe OR "nivel de escritura" OR "writing ability" OR "capacité d'écriture" OR schreibfähigkeit OR "capacidad de escritura" OR "writing skills" OR "compétences en écriture" OR schreibfertigkeiten OR "habilidades de escritura" OR numeracy OR analphabetism OR calcul OR rechnen OR aritmética OR cálculo OR "health education" OR "éducation sanitaire" OR "éducation sur la santé" OR Gesundheitserziehung OR "educación para la salud" OR "health knowledge" OR "connaissances sur la santé" OR Gesundheitswissen OR "conocimientos sobre la salud" OR attitude* OR Einstellungen OR Actitudes OR "health adj" OR competenc* OR competence OR capacité OR Kompetenz OR competencia OR "health communication" OR "communication sur la santé" OR Gesundheitskommunikation OR "comunicación en salud" OR "patient education" OR "éducation du patient" OR Patientenaufklärung OR Patientenerziehung OR "educación del paciente"	Title/ abstract

Table A1.1. Search strategy in English, French, German and Spanish (contd)

	Terms	Type
AND	Evaluation OR évaluation OR Evaluierung OR evaluación OR measure OR mesure OR messen OR medida OR assessment OR évaluation OR analyse OR Bewertung OR evaluación OR análisis OR screening OR dépistage OR selection OR cribado OR instrument OR instrument OR instrument OR questionnaire OR sondage OR Fragebogen OR cuestionario OR encuesta OR outcome OR résultat OR Ergebnis OR resultado OR thematic OR thématique OR thematisch OR temático OR logic* OR Logique OR Logik OR lógica OR measurement OR mesure OR Messung OR medición OR evidence OR preuve OR Beweise OR evidencia OR framework OR cadre OR Rahmen OR marco de referencia OR model OR modèle OR Modell OR modelo OR tool OR outil OR Werkzeug OR herramienta OR resource OR Ressource OR recurso OR domain* OR Domäne OR dominio OR scale OR échelle OR Masstab OR Skala OR escala OR dashboard OR "tableau de bord" OR Instrumententafel OR salpicadero OR "case study" OR "étude de cas" OR Fallstudie OR "estudio de caso" OR indicator* OR indicateur OR Indikator OR indicador OR measure* OR qualitative OR qualitative OR cualitativ*	Title/ abstract
AND	Patient OR paciente OR person OR personne OR persona OR individual OR Individuel OR Individuell OR consumer OR consommatrice OR consommateur OR Verbraucher OR consumidor OR citizen OR citoyen OR Bürger OR ciudadano OR community OR communauté OR Gemeinschaft OR comunidad OR public OR Publique OR öffentlich OR Öffentlichkeit OR público OR población OR "distributed" distribué* OR verteilt OR repartido OR distribuido OR policy OR politique OR Politik OR política OR system OR système OR sistema OR education OR éducation OR Bildung OR educación OR formación OR school OR école OR Schule OR colegio OR escuela OR workplace OR "lieu de travail" OR Arbeitsplatz OR "lugar de trabajo" OR employment OR emploi OR Beschäftigung OR empleo OR digital OR numérique OR digitale OR numérico OR environment OR Umwelt OR "medio ambiente" OR media OR medias OR Medien OR "medios de comunicación" OR "mass media"	Title/ abstract

Table A1.1. Search strategy in English, French, German and Spanish (contd)

	Terms	Type
AND	policy OR politique OR Politik OR política OR intervention OR intervención OR "Health promotion" OR "promotion de la santé" OR Gesundheitsförderung OR "intervention study" OR "étude d'intervention" OR Interventionsstudie OR "estudio de intervención" OR "Government Programmes" OR "programme gouvernemental" OR Regierungsprogramm OR "programa gubernamental" OR program* OR effect* OR "intervention studies"	Title/ abstract
AND	English OR French OR German OR Spanish OR Russian	Language
NOT	Editorial OR éditorial OR redaktionell OR letter OR lettre OR Brief OR carta OR comment OR commentaire OR Kommentar OR comentario	Publication type
NOT	dyslectic OR dyslexi* OR dyslectique OR dyslektisch OR disléxico OR "Dyslexia" OR dyslexie OR dislexia	Title/ abstract

Table A1.2. Search strategy in Russian

	Термины (terms)	тип (type)
	грамотность в вопросах здоровья (literacy in questions of health) ИЛИ (OR) грамотн* здоровь* (literacy health) ИЛИ мед* грамотн* (medical literacy) ИЛИ мед* информированн* (medical awareness) ИЛИ медицин* активн* (medical activity)	All fields
ИЛИ (OR)	Знани* (knowledge) ИЛИ отношени* (attitude) ИЛИ навык* (skills) ИЛИ обучени*(education) ИЛИ активност* (activity) ИЛИ информированн* (awareness) ИЛИ информаци* (information) ИЛИ компетенци* (competence) ИЛИ осведомленн* (awareness)	Название/ аннотация (title/abstract)

Table A1.2. Search strategy in Russian (contd)

	Термины (terms)	тип (type)
И (AND)	Измерение (measurement) ИЛИ оценка (assessment/estimation) ИЛИ анализ (analysis) ИЛИ анкета (questionnaire) ИЛИ программа (programme)	Название/ аннотация (title/abstract)
И (AND)	Пациент (patient) ИЛИ молодежь (young people) ИЛИ население (population) ИЛИ система (system) ИЛИ образование (education) ИЛИ школа (school) ИЛИ рабочее место (workplace) ИЛИ образ жизни (lifestyle)	Название/ аннотация (title/abstract)
И (AND)	Политика (policy) ИЛИ программа (programme) ИЛИ мера (measure) ИЛИ вмешательство (intervention)	Название/ аннотация (title/abstract)
И (AND)	Russian	язык (language)
НЕ (NOT)	Редакционное письмо ИЛИ письмо ИЛИ комментарий (editorial OR letter OR comment)	Тип публикации (publication type)
НЕ (NOT)	дислексия dyslexia	Название/ аннотация (title/abstract)

Data extraction

The identified studies were analysed using a synthesis framework based on the Ladder of Measurement (2), and guided by the project steering group. The framework contained the following criteria for data extraction: conceptual frameworks, logic models, methods, data sources, indicators, governance, partnerships, outputs and validated tools. The validated tools were further described by which aspects of health literacy they measured (functional, interactive, critical, distributed, public or organizational), societal areas and levels, and whether they measured absolute skills (test-based) or perceived skills (self-reported). The geographical range of the studies (international, regional, national or local) was also recorded. Figs A1.1–A1.3 show the selection process for the final 81 documents.

Fig. A1.1. Selection of studies in English, French, German and Spanish

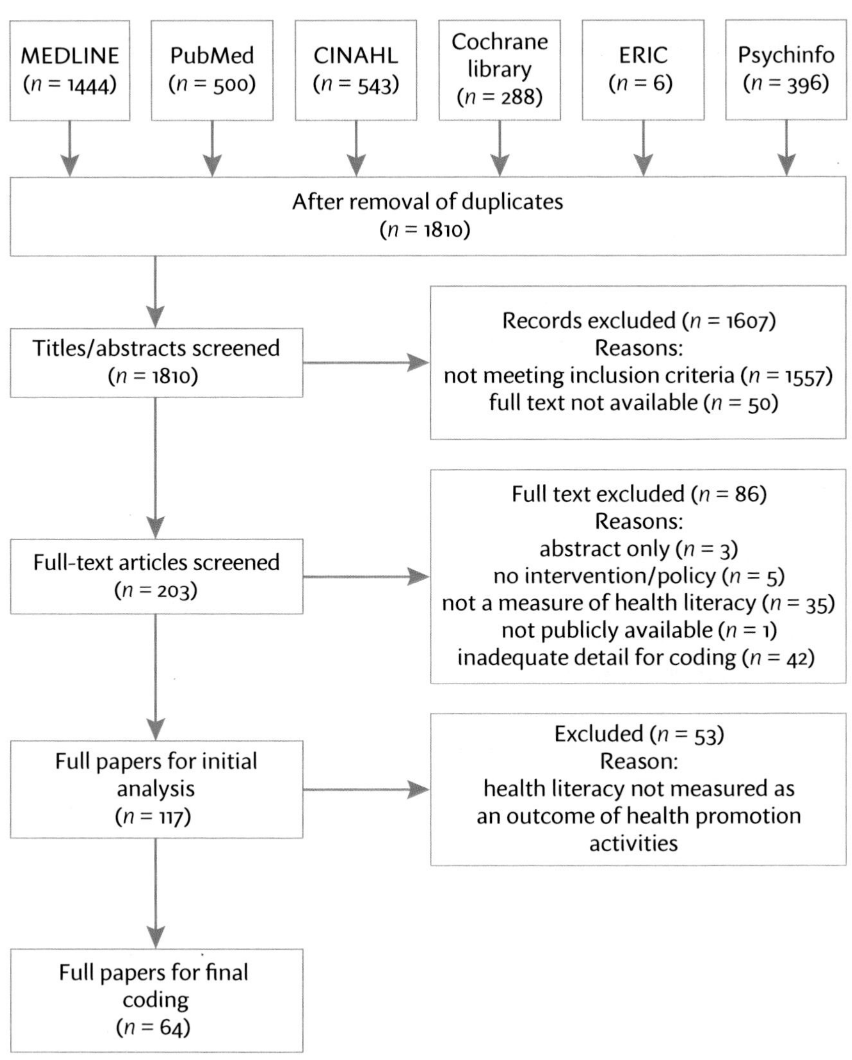

Fig. A1.2. Selection of studies in Russian

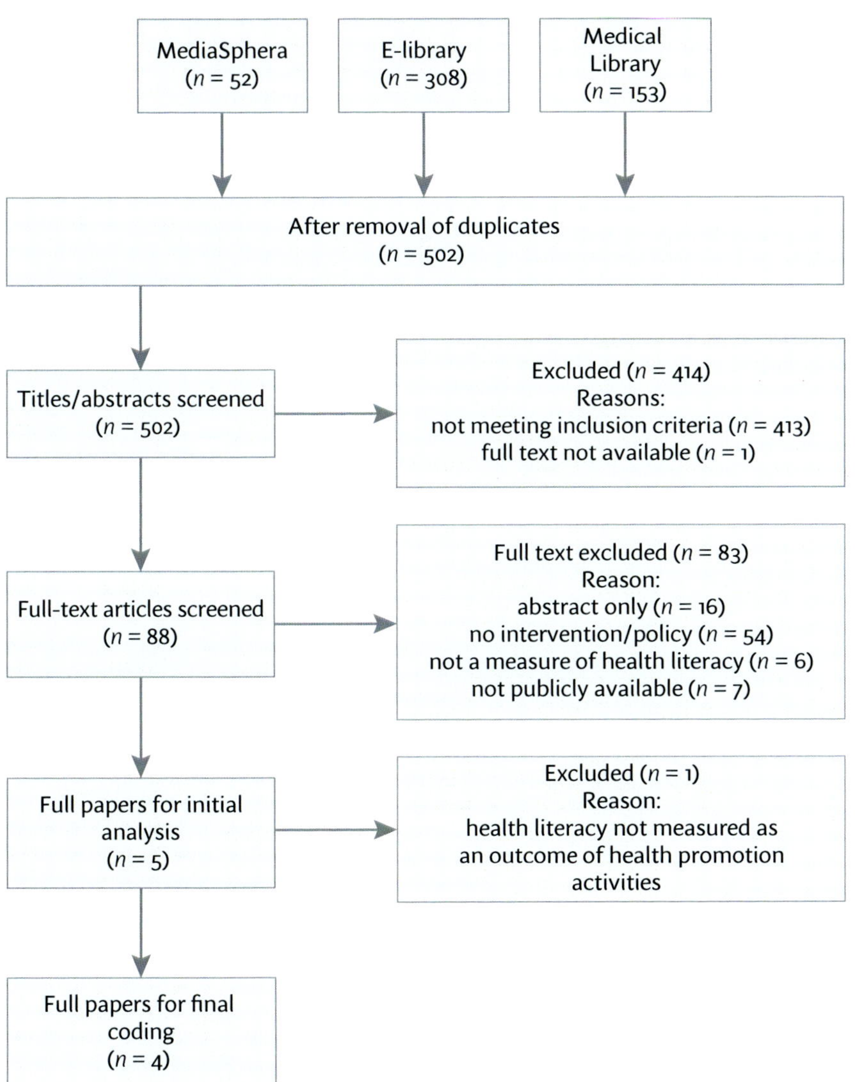

Fig. A1.3. Combined search results

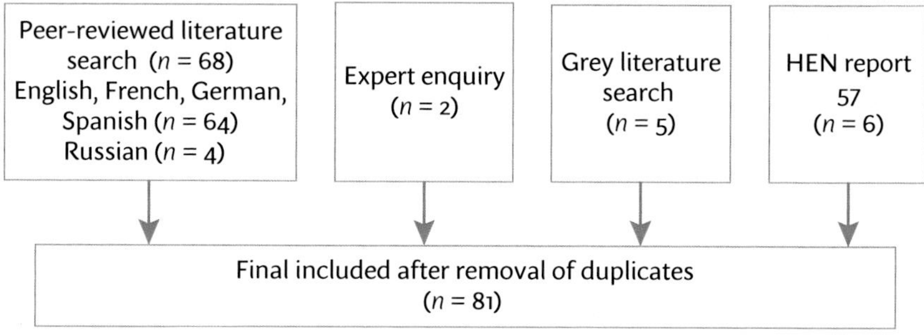

References

1. Rowlands G, Russell S, O'Donnell A, Kaner E, Trezona A, Rademakers J et al. What is the evidence on existing policies and linked activities and their effectiveness for improving health literacy at national, regional and organizational levels in the WHO European Region? Copenhagen: WHO Regional Office for Europe; 2018 (Health Evidence Network (HEN) synthesis report 57; http://www.euro.who.int/__data/assets/pdf_file/0006/373614/Health-evidence-network-synthesis-WHO-HEN-Report-57.pdf?ua=1, accessed 10 August 2019).

2. Rippon S, South J. Promoting asset based approaches for health and well-being: exploring a theory of change and challenges in evaluation. Leeds: Leeds Beckett University; 2017 (http://eprints.leedsbeckett.ac.uk/4497/7/Promoting%20asset%20based%20approaches%20Nov%202017.pdf, accessed 10 August 2019).

ANNEX 2. RELEVANT HEALTH LITERACY CONCEPTS

Multiple concepts and definitions have emerged as research into health literacy has developed. This section is not a comprehensive overview of the topic, which is covered in depth elsewhere (1). Rather it aims to illustrate how the conceptual paradigm within which a health literacy measurement or evaluation is sited will influence the settings for the studies and activities, the frameworks and logic models applied and the indicators chosen and measured.

Clinical (or medical) perspectives

Clinical (or medical) perspectives of health literacy are characterized by a focus on the literacy, language and numeracy skills required by individuals to perform tasks within a health-care environment, and on the skills of those providing health services to tailor services to patient health literacy needs (2,3). Measurement and evaluation activities with this clinical perspective will usually take place in medical settings and will focus on specific medical conditions. Outcomes of health literacy activities might include improved access to health care, strengthened patient–provider interactions and communication, improved patient compliance with recommended treatment, enhanced patients' capacity to manage their own health, and improved health (4); these outcomes will be reflected in the indicators of change and the tools used to measure any change.

Public health perspectives

Public health perspectives are underpinned by principles of participation, social justice and equity. Health literacy is viewed as an asset that can be built through community empowerment, civic engagement and social action (4,5), as well as a determinant of health. Within this paradigm, health literacy involves capacities to actively participate in health and health-related activities and to exert greater control over life events and situations (6). Health literacy measurement and evaluation with a public health perspective may, consequently, take place in a wide range of settings: "Health is created and lived by people within the settings of their everyday life; where they learn, work, play and love" (7). Outcomes, and hence indicators and measurement tools, will vary according to the setting and the focus of the activity but could include personal knowledge and capability, skills in negotiation and self-management, skills in social organization and advocacy, health literacy (skills and capabilities), changed health behaviours and practices, engagement in social actions for health, participation in changing social norms and practices, and improved health and increased opportunities for health and well-being (6).

Organizational perspectives

Organizational health literacy models and frameworks focus on the relationship between the health literacy skills of individuals and the complexity of health services and systems. These models have been developed to emphasize the responsibility of health and social care organizations to reduce the health literacy demands they place on people. They also provide guidance on the actions that organizations need to take to improve the way they respond to the health literacy needs of service users. Examples of organizational health literacy frameworks include the Institute of Medicine's Ten Attributes Model (8), the Organisational Health Literacy Responsiveness Framework (9) and the Vienna Health Literate Organisation model (10). The domains contained within these frameworks broadly include: (i) leadership, management and organizational culture; (ii) systems and processes; (iii) planning and evaluation; (iv) consumer consultation, engagement and partnerships; (v) workforce; (vi) access and navigation; and (vii) communication practices and principles.

Specific aspects of personal health literacy

As a consequence of the trend in health literacy to use the terms health and literacy in a more comprehensive way, definitions and measures have evolved for specific aspects of personal health literacy (e.g. different age groups; different lifestyles; specific diseases; specific aspects of health; and in relation to specific types of communication such as oral, written or digital) (11). Two examples of this are given.

Digital health literacy. This concept is attracting increasing focus because of the advances in digital technology and its potential as an important method of communication of information to "make judgements and take decisions (for health) in everyday life" (1). A widely used definition states that digital health literacy is "the ability to seek, find, understand, and appraise health information from electronic sources and apply the knowledge gained to addressing or solving a health problem" (12).

Mental health literacy. This concept has developed separately from the wider health literacy field. Early definitions focused on peoples' knowledge, attitudes and beliefs about mental disorders that would aid their recognition, management or prevention (13). As in the wider health literacy field, the definition has evolved to include the skills to obtain and maintain positive mental health and to seek mental health help when needed (14). The outcomes of mental health literacy activities, and hence the indicators of change studied and the tools used to demonstrate that change, may vary widely according to the definition of mental health literacy that the particular study is using. Some studies will focus solely on knowledge, attitudes and beliefs about mental health, while others will include elements of mental health capacities.

References

1. Sørensen K, Van den Broucke S, Fullam J, Doyle G, Pelikan J, Slonska Z et al. Health literacy and public health: a systematic review and integration of definitions and models. BMC Public Health. 2012;12:80. doi: 10.1186/1471-2458-12-80.
2. Mancuso JM. Assessment and measurement of health literacy: an integrative review of the literature. Nurs Health Sci. 2009;11(1):77–89. doi: 10.1111/j.1442-2018.2008.00408.x.
3. Paasche-Orlow MK, Wolf MS. The causal pathways linking health literacy with health outcomes. Am J Health Behav. 2007;31(suppl 1):S19–26. doi: 10.5555/ajhb.2007.31.supp.S19.
4. Nutbeam D. Health literacy as a public health goal: a challenge for contemporary health education and communication strategies into the 21st century. Health Promot Int. 2000;15(3):259–67. doi: 10.1080/10810730.2017.1417515.
5. Freedman DA, Bess KD, Tucker HA, Boyd DL, Tuchman AM, Wallston KA. Public health literacy defined. Am J Prev Med. 2009;36(5):446–51. doi: 10.1016/j.amepre.2009.02.001.
6. Nutbeam D. The evolving concept of health literacy. Soc Sci Med. 2008;67(12):2072–8. doi: 10.1016/j.socscimed.2008.09.050.
7. Ottawa charter for health promotion. Geneva: World Health Organization; 1986 (http://www.euro.who.int/__data/assets/pdf_file/0004/129532/Ottawa_Charter.pdf?ua=1, accessed 13 August 2019).
8. Brach C, Keller D, Hernandez LM, Baur C, Parker R, Dreyer B et al. Ten attributes of health literate health care organizations; a discussion paper. Washington (DC): Institute of Medicine; 2012.

9. Trezona A, Dodson S, Osborne RH. Development of the Organisational Health Literacy Responsiveness (Org-HLR) self-assessment tool and process. BMC Health Serv Res. 2018;18(1):694. doi: 10.1186/s12913-018-3499-6.

10. Dietscher C, Pelikan JM. Health literate hospitals and healthcare organizations: results from an Austrian feasibility study on the self-assessment of organizational health literacy in hospitals. In: Schaeffer D, Pelikan JM, editors. Health literacy: Forschungsstand und Perspektiven. Gottingen: Hogrefe; 2017:303–14.

11. Pelikan JM, Ganahl K. Measuring health literacy in general populations: primary findings from the HLS-EU Consortium's health literacy assessment effort. In: Logan RA, Sigel ER, editors. Health literacy. Amsterdam: IOS Press; 2017:34–59.

12. Norman CD, Skinner HA. eHealth literacy: essential skills for consumer health in a networked world. J Med Internet Res. 2006;8(2):e9. doi: 10.2196/jmir.8.2.e9.

13. Jorm AF, Korten AE, Jacomb PA, Christensen H, Rodgers B, Pollitt P. „Mental health literacy": a survey of the public's ability to recognise mental disorders and their beliefs about the effectiveness of treatment. Med J Aust. 1997;166(4):182–6. doi: 10.5555/ajhb.2007.31.supp.S19.

14. Kutcher S, Bagnell A, Wei Y. Mental health literacy in secondary schools: a Canadian approach. Child Adolesc Psychiatr Clin N Am. 2015;24(2):233–44. doi: 10.1016/j.chc.2014.11.007.

ANNEX 3. CHARACTERISTICS OF HEALTH LITERACY INSTRUMENTS

Table A3.1. Characteristics of health literacy instruments

Instrument	Acronym	Assessment type[a]	Domains/scales	Validated
Personal health literacy for general populations				
All Aspects of Health Literacy Scale (1)	AAHLS[b]	Self-report	(i) Functional HL, (ii) interactive HL, (iii) critical HL, (iv) empowerment	Y
Communicative and Critical Health Literacy Scale (2)	C&CHL	Self-report	(i) Communicative HL, (ii) critical HL	Y
Health Literacy Questionnaire (3)	HLQ	Self-report	(i) Feel understood and supported by health-care providers, (ii) have sufficient information to manage my health, (iii) actively manage my health, (iv) social support for health, (v) appraisal of health information, (vi) ability to actively engage with health-care providers, (vii) able to navigate the health-care system, (viii) ability to find good health information, (ix) understand health information well enough to know what to do	Y
Health Literacy Scale (4)	HLS-14	Self-report	(i) Functional HL, (ii) communicative HL, (iii) critical HL	Y

Table A3.1. Characteristics of health literacy instruments (contd)

Instrument	Acronym	Assessment type[a]	Domains/scales	Validated
European Health Literacy Questionnaire 47 (5)	HLS-EUQ47[b]	Self-report	(i) Access/obtain information, (ii) understand information relevant to health, (iii) process/appraise information relevant to health, (iv) apply/use information relevant to health (across health care, disease prevention, health promotion)	Y
European Health Literacy Questionnaire 16 (6)	HLS-EUQ16	Self-report	(i) Access/obtain information, (ii) understand information relevant to health, (iii) process/appraise information relevant to health, (iv) apply/use information relevant to health (across health care, disease prevention, health promotion)	Y
Rapid Estimate of Health Literacy in Medicine (7)	REALM	Test-based	Reading	Y
Single Item Literacy Screener (8)	SILS	Self-report	Reading	Y
Personal health literacy for specific populations				
Health Literacy for School-aged Children Instrument (9)	HLSAC[b]	Self-report	(i) Theoretical knowledge, (ii) practical knowledge, (iii) critical thinking, (iv) self-awareness, (v) citizenship	Y
Short Test of Functional Health Literacy in Adults (10)	STOFHLA[b]	Test-based	Functional HL (numeracy, reading, comprehension)	Y

Table A3.1. Characteristics of health literacy instruments (contd)

Instrument	Acronym	Assessment type[a]	Domains/scales	Validated
Test of Functional Health Literacy in Adults (11)	TOFHLA	Test-based	Functional HL (numeracy, reading, comprehension)	Y
Digital health literacy				
Digital Health Literacy Assessment Tool (12)	DHLAT	Open-ended	(i) Access information, (ii) understand information, (iii) process/appraise information, (iv) apply/use information	N
e-Health Literacy Scale (13)	eHEALS	Self-report	(i) Knowledge, (ii) skills, (iii) confidence	Y
Condition- or topic-specific health literacy				
Critical Nutrition Literacy Instrument (14)	CNLI[b]	Self-report	(i) Engagement in dietary habits, (ii) take a critical stance towards nutrition scales and their sources	Y
Diabetes Health Literacy Survey (15)	DHLS	Test-based	(i) Type 2 diabetes information, (ii) clinical management information, (iii) self-management, (iv) ethnomedical (cultural) beliefs	N
High Blood Pressure Health Literacy Scale (16)	HBP HLS	Test-based	(i) Print literacy (reading/ comprehension), (ii) functional HL (numeracy)	Y
Ishikawa Health Literacy Survey (17)	–	Self-report	(i) Functional HL, (ii) communicative (interactive) HL, (iii) critical HL	Y
Malaria Health Literacy Questionnaire (18)	–	Test-based, self-report	(i) Knowledge, (ii) attitudes, (iii) practices, (iv) skills	Y

Table A3.1. Characteristics of health literacy instruments (contd)

Instrument	Acronym	Assessment type[a]	Domains/scales	Validated
Oral Health Literacy Instrument (19)	OHLI	Test-based	(i) Reading (comprehension), (ii) numeracy	Y
Rapid Estimate of Health Literacy in Dentistry (short form) (20)	REALD-30	Test-based	Reading	Y
Smoking Media Literacy Scale (21)	SML	Self-report	(i) Authors and audiences, (ii) messages and meanings, (iii) representation and reality (understanding and appraisal across the three domains)	Y
Organizational health literacy (responsiveness)				
Health Literacy Assessment Questions (for health-care providers) (22)	HLAQ	Self-report	(i) Communication skills, (ii) patient–provider collaboration, (iii) support of patients	N
HeLLO Tas!: a toolkit for health literacy learning organizations (23)	HeLLO Tas!	Self-report	(i) Consumer involvement, (ii) workforce, (iii) meeting the needs of diverse communities, (iv) access and navigation, (v) communication, (vi) leadership and management	N
Mental health literacy				
Anxiety Literacy Scale (24)	A-Lit	Test-based	Knowledge	Y

Table A3.1. Characteristics of health literacy instruments (contd)

Instrument	Acronym	Assessment type[a]	Domains/scales	Validated
Adolescent Depression Knowledge Questionnaire (25)	ADKQ	Test-based	Knowledge	Y
Depression Literacy Scale (26)	D-Lit	Test-based	Knowledge	Y
Mental Health Knowledge Scale (27)	MAKS[b]	Self-report	Knowledge (stigma and conditions)	Y
Mental Health Knowledge and Attitudes Scale (28)	MHKAS	Self-report and test-based	(i) Knowledge, (ii) attitudes	N
Mental Health Literacy Scale (29)	MHLS[b]	Self-report and test-based	(i) Knowledge, (ii) attitudes	Y
Mental Health Literacy Tool for the Workplace (30)	MHL-W	Self-report	(i) Knowledge, (ii) confidence, (iii) attitudes	Y
Mental Health Literacy Questionnaire (31)	MHLQ	Self-report and test-based	(i) Knowledge (identification), (ii) beliefs, (iii) attitudes	N

Notes: HL: health literacy; N: no; Y: yes.

[a]Test-based measures refer to performance-measuring objective tests (where the result is correct or incorrect) and describes absolute skills not related to context/environment; self-report measures refers to individual perceptions about their own health literacy (where the result is reported on a scale), which will reflect the balance between skills and context/environment.

[b]Shows instruments used in studies conducted in the WHO European Region.

References

1. Chinn D, McCarthy C. All Aspects of Health Literacy Scale (AAHLS): developing a tool to measure functional, communicative and critical health literacy in primary healthcare settings. Patient Educ Couns. 2013;90(2):247–53. doi: 10.1016/j.pec.2012.10.019.
2. Ishikawa H, Nomura K, Sato M, Yano E. Developing a measure of communicative and critical health literacy: a pilot study of Japanese office workers. Health Promot Int. 2008;23(3):269–74. doi: 10.1093/heapro/dan017.
3. Osborne RH, Batterham RW, Elsworth GR, Hawkins M, Buchbinder R. The grounded psychometric development and initial validation of the Health Literacy Questionnaire (HLQ). BMC Public Health. 2013;13:658. doi: 10.1186/1471-2458-13-658.
4. Suka M, Odajima T, Kasai M. The 14-item health literacy scale for Japanese adults (HLS-14). Environ Health Prev Med. 2013;18(5):407–15. doi: 10.1007/s12199-013-0340-z.
5. Sørensen K, Van den Broucke S, Pelikan JM, Fullam J, Doyle G, Slonska Z et al. Measuring health literacy in populations: illuminating the design and development process of the European Health Literacy Survey Questionnaire (HLS-EU-Q). BMC Public Health. 2013;13:948. doi: 10.1186/1471-2458-13-948.
6. Sørensen K, Pelikan JM, Rothlin F, Ganahl K, Slonska Z, Doyle G et al. Health literacy in Europe: comparative results of the European health literacy survey (HLS-EU). Eur J Public Health. 2015;25(6):1053–8. doi: 10.1093/eurpub/ckv043.
7. Davis TC, Crouch MA, Long SW, Jackson RH, Bates P, George RB et al. Rapid assessment of literacy levels of adult primary care patients. Fam Med. 1991;23(6):433–5. PMID: 1936717
8. Morris N, MacLean CD, Chew LD, Littenberg B. The single item literacy screener: evaluation of a brief instrument to identify limited reading ability. BMC Fam Pract. 2006;7:21–7.
9. Paakkari O, Torppa M, Kannas L, Paakkari L. Subjective health literacy: development of a brief instrument for school-aged children. Scand J Public Health. 2016;44(8):751–7. doi: 10.1177/1403494816669639.
10. Baker DW, Williams MV, Parker RM, Gazmararian JA, Nurss J. Development of a brief test to measure functional health literacy. Patient Educ Couns. 1999;38(1):33–42. PMID: 14528569.

11. Parker RM, Baker DW, Williams MV, Nurss JR. The test of functional health literacy in adults: a new instrument for measuring patients' literacy skills. J Gen Intern Med. 1995;10(10):537–41. doi: 10.1007/bf02640361.

12. St Jean B, Greene Taylor N, Kodama C, Subramaniam M. Assessing the digital health literacy skills of tween participants in a school-library-based after-school program. J Consum Health Internet. 2017;21(1):40–61. doi 10.1080/15398285.2017.1279894.

13. Chung S, Nahm ES. Testing reliability and validity of the eHealth Literacy Scale (eHEALS) for older adults recruited online. Comput Inform Nurs. 2015;33(4):150–6. doi: 10.1097/CIN.0000000000000146.

14. Guttersrud O, Dalane J, Pettersen S. Improving measurement in nutrition literacy research using Rasch modelling: examining construct validity of stage-specific "critical nutrition literacy" scales. Public Health Nutr. 2014;17(4):877–83. doi: 10.1017/S1368980013000530.

15. Calderón JL, Shaheen M, Hays RD, Fleming ES, Norris KC, Baker RS. Improving diabetes health literacy by animation. Diabetes Educ. 2014;40(3):361–72. doi: 10.1177/0145721714527518.

16. Kim MT, Song HJ, Han HR, Song Y, Nam S, Nguyen TH et al. Development and validation of the high blood pressure-focused health literacy scale. Patient Educ Couns. 2012;87(2):165–70. doi: 10.1016/j.pec.2011.09.005.

17. Ishikawa H, Takeuchi T, Yano E. Measuring functional, communicative, and critical health literacy among diabetic patients. Diabetes Care. 2008;31(5):874–9. doi: 10.2337/dc07-1932.

18. Li W, Han LQ, Guo YJ, Sun J. Using WeChat official accounts to improve malaria health literacy among Chinese expatriates in Niger: an intervention study. Malar J. 2016;15(1):567. doi: 10.1186/s12936-016-1621-y.

19. Sabbahi DA, Lawrence HP, Limeback H. Development and evaluation of an oral health literacy instrument for adults. Community Dent Oral Epidemiol. 2009;37(5):451–62. doi: 10.1111/j.1600-0528.2009.00490.x.

20. Lee J, Rozier R, Lee S, Bender D, Ruiz R. Development of a word recognition instrument to test health literacy in dentistry: the REALD-30 – a brief communication. J Public Health Dent. 2007;67(2):94–8. PMID: 17557680.

21. Primack BA, Gold MA, Switzer GE, Hobbs R, Land SR, Fine MJ. Development and validation of a smoking media literacy scale for adolescents. Arch Pediatr Adolesc Med. 2006;160(4):369–74. doi: 10.1001/archpedi.160.4.369.

22. Cooper J, Davenport M, Gaillard K, Kompier A. Health literacy in practice program evaluation. Kalamazoo (MI): School of Social Work, Western Michigan University; 2011.

23. HELLO TAS! toolkit (a toolkit for health literacy learning organisations). Sandy Bay: Tasmanian Council of Social Services; 2019 (https://www.hellotas.org.au, accessed 12 August 2019).

24. Gulliver A, Griffiths KM, Christensen H, Mackinnon A, Calear AL, Parsons A et al. Internet-based interventions to promote mental health help-seeking in elite athletes: an exploratory randomized controlled trial. J Med Internet Res. 2012;14(3):e69. doi: 10.2196/jmir.1864.

25. Hart SR, Kastelic EA, Wilcox HC. Achieving depression literacy: the Adolescent Depression Knowledge Questionnaire. School Ment Health. 2014;6(3):213–23. doi: 10.1007/s12310-014-9120-1.

26. Griffiths KM, Christensen H, Jorm AF, Evans K, Groves C. Effect of web-based depression literacy and cognitive-behavioural therapy interventions on stigmatising attitudes to depression: randomised controlled trial. Br J Psychiatry. 2004;185:342–9. doi: 10.1192/bjp.185.4.342.

27. Evans-Lacko S, Little K, Meltzer H, Rose D, Rhydderch D, Henderson C et al. Development and psychometric properties of the Mental Health Knowledge Schedule. Can J Psychiatry. 2010;55(7):440–8. doi: 10.1177/070674371005500707.

28. Kutcher S, Wei Y. Educator mental health literacy: a programme evaluation of the teacher training education on the mental health & high school curriculum guide. Adv Sch Ment Health Promot. 2013;6(2):83–92. doi: https://doi.org/10.1080/1754730X.2013.784615.

29. O'Connor M, Casey L. The Mental Health Literacy Scale (MHLS): a new scale-based measure of mental health literacy. Psychiatry Res. 2015;229(1–2):511–16. doi: 10.1016/j.psychres.2015.05.064.

30. Moll S, Zanhour M, Patten S, Stuart H, MacDermid J. Evaluating mental health literacy in the workplace: development and psychometric properties of a vignette-based tool. J Occup Rehabil. 2017;27(4):601–11. doi: 10.1007/s10926-017-9695-0.

31. Reavley NJ, Jorm AF. National survey of mental health literacy and stigma. Canberra: Department of Health and Ageing; 2011.